D1518441

Pills, Bills, & Parkinson's Disease

Coping with the On-Off Syndrome

by
Paul A. Luscombe

Contents

Acknowledgments

Upon completion of my book *Howard Powerless*, my will to write another book was somewhat dampened by the effort it took to finally piece together all the loose ends at the conclusion of the project. I sincerely wanted to write, but as my Parkinson's factor intensified, I realized I would become more dependent on others to get something meaningful into publication. Thus, I shifted gears and decided to focus on my own personal experiences as a Parkinson's victim. Research would be minimal, interviews with others would not be essential, I could start immediately, and the more I investigated, the more I came to the conclusion that the need for such a book might be substantial.

When I mentioned my idea to my two neurologists, both—Dr. Cheryl Waters of Columbia University's Neurological Institute and Dr. Melvin Vigman of Summit, New Jersey—were very enthusiastic about such a project. They were 100 percent behind my effort and basically told me to "go for it." Dr. Waters agreed to write a short Foreword for the piece. Dr. Vigman had followed my case since my first appointment on February 18, 1992, when he broke the news to me that he felt I was stricken with PD.

Inside this book, I jokingly refer to members of the Chatham Men's Club. My college pal Doug Hobby is the mainstay of the group. He drives me short distances to destinations such as the post office, and we also go on longer trips like our journey to see the Lafayette College versus Delaware University football game. I recall calling Doug (an engineering major at Lafayette) at three a.m. when our basement flooded last summer, and he was over in a matter of minutes. Whenever I'm able to participate in golf tournaments and outings, Doug is usually my partner. If it weren't for Doug, I would have given up golf long ago!

Raymond Monroe and Kelly Dodson, both of Florida, have stayed at our home for extended visits and have been very helpful to my wife with respect to chores more traditionally filled by "the man of the house." Raymond and Kelly were also the most ambitious about playing card games (such as Skip BO) and other intellectually challenging games. Both encourage me to stick with my therapy programs, to participate in as many outside activities as possible, and to remain fundamentally positive throughout my adversity. A day with Raymond and/or Kelly seems to fly by very quickly.

My next-door neighbor Ken Thompson, who works for the Securitas Corporation, has an irregular work schedule, but we frequently have lunch together at Hooters restaurant on Route 22 in Union, New Jersey. On the occasion of a major sporting event, such as a New York JETS football game, Ken facilitates a meeting of the Men's Club and we may watch the event in my living room or we may hold our meeting at O'Reilly's Pub in Maplewood, New Jersey. Sometimes we are joined by Doug's son Brian. Other lunch partners include Bob Faig and Vin Morris.

My family has also been highly supportive and active in easing the discomfort of PD. My wife is definitely not a morning person, but she has been like a saint in helping me get started with my day. She maintains a very active work schedule with her position at the Paper Mill Playhouse, and she is in constant motion as she gets my day organized before she leaves for work. Our two daughters—Alison and Priscilla—live a distance from Chatham, but both offer constant encouragement via e-mail messages and telephone calls.

The newest member of our family is my son-in-law Erik Swift, who edited several of the chapters and constantly has tried to include me in his active social life.

Finally, I wish to cite the role of Janet Reno, former attorney general of the United States during the Clinton Administration. Her fulfillment of the rigors of this position, coupled with her own PD problems, were an inspiration to me. I also was impressed by her run for the Florida governor's office in 2002. In April of 2005, I had the opportunity to meet with her during our vacation in Key Biscayne, Florida. When I mentioned that she inspired me, she mentioned that I inspired her! Our meeting closed with Reno saying: "For Paul: Thank you for inspiring us all with your strength, courage and humor." At the end of our meeting, she insisted on a big hug!

Foreword

By Dr. Cheryl H. Waters,
Albert B. and Judith L. Glickman Professor,
Chief of Clinical Practice and Services,
Neurological Institute of New York,
Columbia University,
Center for Parkinson's Disease &
Other Movement Disorders

Most of the books written about Parkinson's disease are authored from the technical side, by doctors and specialists working within the field of Neurology. When my patient Paul Luscombe asked me what I thought about a book written by a Parkinson's victim about his everyday experiences and coping with life in general, I was quite enthusiastic about the prospects for a meaningful book. Also, I knew Paul was an accomplished author, and had three books in publication. He also was very conscientious about writing me personal memos in advance of his appointments at Columbia. Also, Paul participated in two of our clinical research projects and his observations were very helpful to my staff. At the time of this publication, he was just starting a third research project to test a new drug.

To the extent that his book alleviates some of the discomfort and suffering from Parkinson's disease, it has served a meaningful purpose. Some of the practical solutions he has suggested, such as substituting a coffee mug for a shallow but elegant soup dish at his daughter's wedding reception, are simple yet functional alternatives to potentially embarrassing situations.

Although Paul's business career on Wall Street was cut short by the ravages of PD, he was able to capitalize on his innate writing ability and formed the PAL Publishing Company to serve as a conduit for his writings. Paul's message of maintaining a purpose in life and remaining continually active are well documented. His pursuit of friendships on a broad basis has helped him constantly in participating in many events that otherwise would not have been possible. Despite the degenerative effect of PD, Paul is always seeking some form of self-improvement. Paul is a survivor.

If you have PD or have a loved one or a friend who has Parkinson's, you should read this book to foster a better understanding of the disease. Not only will you obtain a better grasp of what he or she goes through on a daily basis, but also you might be entertained as well! Paul's is not a joyful adjustment process, as he illustrates in his chapter on sleeping difficulties, but he does inject a sense of humor while trying to maintain an element of reality. Actually, Paul is a very entertaining writer, and his material reads rather effortlessly. Read the book *Pills, Bills, & Parkinson's Disease: Coping with the On-Off Syndrome* by Paul A. Luscombe. You won't be disappointed.

Perhaps I wore out my brain by trying to memorize so many sports statistics!

Chapter 1

General Introduction

In the summer of 1964, more than forty years ago, I was just launching my business career as a bond salesman on Wall Street. Among my early achievements was my selection for membership in the Bond Club of New Jersey, a professional society consisting of approximately 250 bankers and stock or bond personnel working in the Garden State. Now, in 2005, I have just completed my second round as a member of the group's board of governors after having served as president for 1976 to 1977 and on the board from 1970 to 1980. I am quite sure that everyone in the club who has met me or knows me is aware that I suffer from Parkinson's disease.

In late September of 2003, I participated in the group's annual Fall Golf Outing at Fairmount Golf Club in Chatham. Upon arriving at the function, I was immediately solicited to partake in the BCNJ 50–50 raffle, which boosts the Club's treasury and helps finance future outings at equally attractive golf courses. Without hesitation, I invested $20 in the raffle and put the tickets in my upper left sport jacket pocket. After a full day on the golf course, at dinner that night, when they called the winning raffle number—worth $830 in hard cash—I thought to myself that it surely sounded familiar. After a few seconds, I was able to extract the ticket from my pocket, and just before the emcee was about to read another number, I shouted out, "I think I've got it!" In my excitement, as I was dashing up to collect my winnings, my lazy right foot just couldn't keep up with its counterpart, and I went sprawling across the ballroom floor. I was quickly helped to my feet by two Bond Club members and as I was awarded the $830, I held the cash high in the air for all to see. Concerned that I might have been seriously hurt, the crowd, which had quickly become silent, suddenly burst into applause and cheers upon spotting the cash. I was indeed embarrassed, but my fellow bond-clubbers comforted me. For many in attendance, this was their first experience with the perils of Parkinsonism.

Actually, the outing was one of my more successful ventures since retiring in 1999. My golf game had improved over the summer, and when I shot a 103 with a 35 handicap, my net score was a 68, which was worthy of second prize in Class B. When the emcee reading off the scores at the dinner that night came to my name, he opted to bring the prize (a pro shop gift certificate worth $75) to my table rather than have me risk another fall.

Actually, the Bond Club of New Jersey was involved when I discovered that I had Parkinson's. On a clear spring evening in 1991, I was playing golf with Jim Carson, a client and fellow member of the BCNJ, at the East Orange Golf Club in Short Hills. Our mission was to play just until dark, and thereby get some practice holes in before the BCNJ outing later in the month. We were literally "moonlighting"!

As we walked the first few fairways, Jim noticed that I had a fairly conspicuous limp. When he questioned me, I assured him that thirty-five years of playing basketball were finally taking their toll. But then he also observed that I was having difficulty retrieving tees and ball-markers from my right pants pocket. My somewhat distorted handwriting, as I posted the scorecard, was another matter. Plus my ability to strike the ball with power and consistency had diminished. Jim was used to seeing me score in the high 80s. Suddenly, I was struggling to break 100. Or worse!

Later that evening, Jim mentioned his observations to his wife Leslie. Her immediate response was that I needed to see a neurologist. At age fifty-four, I was anxious to remedy my ailments and, most important, get my golf game back on track. Like my peers in the bond profession, I wanted to play well in the forthcoming outing. On February 18, 1992, the Carsons' comments led me to the office of Dr. Melvin Vigman, a neurologist in Summit.

Dr. Vigman studied my condition, ran an MRI on my brain, and then broke the news to me gently. He explained to me that I had Parkinson's disease.

I suddenly felt old before my time. Naturally, I was shocked and depressed. The thought of my degenerating physical condition, the specter of becoming a zombie-like critter, and a flood of horrific thoughts crossed my mind. Forget the Bond Club outing. At age fifty-four, I figured I was through as a golfer.

But was I? Soon I would do some research on Parkinson's, and my mindset improved dramatically. I found that Parkinson's disease is not the most lethal ailment imaginable. It is, however, a very annoying affliction, and is extremely persistent, preventing its victims from accomplishing what are normally regarded as routine human functions. It also is frequently socially embarrassing. In their worst phases, people stricken with PD appear totally helpless to do anything related to body movement. Although medical research has made significant strides, the PD factor impacts more than one million Americans and at this point remains without a cure.

When talking about Parkinson's disease, you frequently hear the term *dopamine*. Dopamine is the chemical substance that assists the brain in controlling the body's basic activities such as walking, talking, and moving in general. Those stricken with PD just don't produce enough dopamine. The medication taken to stimulate dopamine production is called levodopa/ carbidopa. Once this medication gets into the brain and starts the dopamine manufacturing process, the patient moves from "off" to "on" and starts to move about more normally. In my case, the benefits of the medication last from about two and a half hours to three hours; then I swing back to the "off" position. "The Big Letdown" occurs as the medicine wears off, and I take another round of medicine to get the dopamine engine running again.

The roll call of Parkinson's victims includes several notable personalities. The late Pope John Paul II's death certificate listed Parkinson's disease, from which he had suffered for more than a decade, as a contributing cause. According to the press, PD had reduced the movement of the Pope's throat muscles. Former Attorney General Janet Reno (see preface to this book), actor Michael J. Fox, "Butch" van Breda Kolff (basketball coach for Bill Bradley, Pete Maravich, and Wilt Chamberlain), and Muhummad Ali are all examples of well

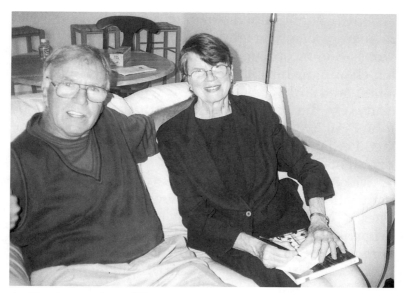

Author Luscombe and former U.S. Attorney General Janet Reno socialize in Key Biscayne, Florida in April 2005. (Photo credit: Anita Weeks)

known Parkinsonians. Also, Adolph Hitler and the late PLO leader Yassir Arafat both suffered from Parkinson's disease.

Is Parkinson's disease hereditary or is it an environmental affliction? Extensive research has yet to yield a conclusive answer to this age-old question. In my situation, I am the only family member on record with the disease. My father and mother both died of cancer and heart-related illnesses. My sister is a healthy specimen at age seventy-four. Also, she has been a tiger in tracking our more distant family members. I believe if she heard that Uncle Harry in Plymouth, Massachusetts had PD, she would verify the fact right away.

Boxer Muhummad Ali (nee Cassius Clay), who reigned as heavyweight champion of the world, provides an interesting example. En route to no less than ten championship fights, Ali must have had his brain jolted on a fairly consistent basis while honing his specialty. On the other hand, as a spiritual leader, Pope John Paul II's life entailed a minimum of physical contact. Perhaps I wore out my brain by trying to memorize so many sports statistics!

Most active Parkinsonians consume numerous medications just to be able to undertake their daily routines.[1] The doctor specializing in neurology sets the original schedule of medication and insists on strict adherence to the plan. Once a distinct pattern emerges, the doctor may allow an element of "pill management" whereby the patient alters the pill schedule to accommodate his/her activities. Doctors insist on authorizing any increase in the number of pills taken.

Because these medications can induce instant drowsiness (i.e., you can't feel the sleepiness coming on), many Parkinsonians do not drive. In fact, during a recent one-on-one luncheon date with Walt Hislop (my key witness for the book I wrote called *Howard Powerless*), I fell asleep while he was talking to me, face-to-face. Embarrassed once again, I had to explain my propensity to fall asleep whenever my body chooses to do so. Ironically, sleeping at night is very difficult because rigidity intensifies while the medications take a breather. In some respects, the bed is my own worst enemy!

---

[1]alternative: form of "brain cell" operation.

In other cases, the dominant outward and visible sign of Parkinson's disease is the phenomenon classi-fied as dyskinesia. *Dyskinesia* is a broad term that refers to the PD victim's excessive but involuntary bodily ac-tivity, especially that of the hands and arms, head, and neck. With most patients, such activity takes place as a result of overstimulation of the dopamines. As the neu-rologists try to fine-tune the proper level of medication, frequently too many pills lead to dyskinesia, and so the doctor may subsequently reduce the future application of the drug therapy. In my own case, I prefer a modest amount of dyskinesia to rigidity.

Many a PD victim must feel like the living example of Sisyphus, the member of Greek mythology con-demned to an eternity of rolling a boulder uphill then watching it roll back down again.

On Versus Off

Most PD patients classify their behavioral patterns into two distinct cycles, simply called "off" and "on." When the PD patient is off, he or she is suffering from the most drastic elements of the disease. These may entail ex-treme rigidity of one's body. In my case, I feel like my body is locked into a vice. If my hand is grasping some object, like a pen or pencil, or even the computer mouse, I have difficulty in releasing until the Parkinson's factor has subsided. In 2005, I had the opportunity to buy a bat-tery operated wheelchair, which would have increased my mobility. But during a week of test runs, I found that my hand could freeze on the forward switch, and I crashed into several walls around our house! We opted to pass on the attractive offer to buy the motorized chair.

While in the off position, I endure immense strain on my legs and knees until I can get a stride going. I find I cannot just start walking, but must have a specific destination in mind before I can move from point A to point B. Excessive "grunting and groaning" may help accomplish a simple task. Basic maneuvers, such as pulling up my trousers, often require outside assistance.

The frustration surrounding PD is created by the need to mentally work out how to accomplish the fundamental body movements of your life, movements which all your life have been second nature but now must be planned in detail. Simple acts, such as placing a telephone bill and a check into the pre-addressed envelope so that the phone company's name and address appear in the envelope window, are frequently impossible or take forever to accomplish. When the patient is on, these actions are easily completed. When off, they are next to impossible to accomplish.[2]

In terms of time, the dichotomy of off and on can be broken down as follows:

Hours in the day: 24
Hours allotted to sleep: 8
   (probably 50% on and 50% off)
Hours awake and allotted: 16
Hours of freeze-ups (off): 4
Hours of normal activity (on): 12

The previous explanation is designed to illustrate my personal experience. In short, I spend some 25 percent

---

[2]To alleviate some of the "envelope anxiety," I have been paying several routine monthly bills by telephone.

of my daytime activity fighting "freeze ups"; the remainder of my non-sleeping time (75%) is spent with "normal activity." This ratio doesn't sound so awful until you incorporate my problems with sleeping in the off position.

Hours in the day: 24
Frozen/off: 8
Normal/on: 12
On hours spent asleep: 4

Thus, I must cram as much activity into those precious hours of on time as I can. To do anything productive entails strict budgeting of my time.*

Believe it or not, in most instances, I have virtually no pain!

Throughout the freeze-ups and dyskinesia, I mostly feel frustration based on my inability to move about freely, and may actually be unaware of any wayward movements of my arms and legs. When sleeping, I may feel very uncomfortable and may search for some time to find a desirable sleeping position.

My freeze-ups vary in intensity and I tend to classify them as Type A, Type B, or Type C. Type A freeze-ups are the worst! They come on extremely strong, sometimes entail a modicum of pain, and last for as long as an hour or two. In many cases, they hit so fast I don't have a chance to anticipate a defensive maneu-

---

*This breakdown reflects my experience with PD after a period of twelve years of treatment and gradually increasing use of PD medicines.

ver. Type A freeze-ups seem to be almost stroke-like in their symptoms. On the other hand, the Type C freeze-up is more common and involves a modest impairment of movement. Type C freeze-ups are the most responsive to the variety of medications that I take. Type B is somewhat of a mixture.

Prescription drugs have evolved as a result of extensive medical research, and they often mitigate the discomforts of PD. As mentioned above, the problems faced due to PD are mainly caused by lack of release of dopamine from the victim's brain. The medicines serve varying roles in releasing these dopamines, and in many cases they can make the PD victim appear "normal" once he or she is in the on cycle. Motor coordination is at its best shortly after the PD medicine kicks in. Usually, the medicine is fairly consistent, but sometimes it takes longer than expected. On rare occasions, a void occurs. In my case, the cycle for on averages about three hours, more or less, and so the "menu" of medicines is generally broken down into three-hour units. Unfortunately, the human body gradually builds an immunity to the various drugs, and so the patient must continually—over time—increase his dosage to accomplish the same results. In my own case, in 1992 I started out taking one sinemet tablet per day; I now take twelve. I also take supportive drugs (comtan, mirapex, and sinemet CR) and hope for relatively normal on periods. At last count, I was taking twenty-two Parkinson's related pills and two prostate pills per day.

External activities, such as appointments or other timely obligations, may cause the patient to "time" his medical intakes so that he or she is at a desirable on position during the event. Another decision is how to handle time zone changes. Some people traveling to different time zones opt to not change pill cycles, while others might make a change to affect a modest improvement in quality of life. For example, in the spring conversion to daylight savings time, the setting of the clocks ahead one hour offers the opportunity to start the day at seven o'clock instead of six. This was appealing to me, because I was able to push my medicines into the more active part of my day. Though adhering to a new time schedule often seems like a good idea, in practice, I tend to slip back to the old schedule.

The victim of Parkinson's disease perpetually lives with one eye on the clock, with his next appointment with his pill supply. Ned Jesser, retired CEO of the United Jersey Banks and a prominent Lafayette College alumnus, was aware of my Parkinson's condition when he invited me to speak before the LC Class of 1939 at their reunion in 2002. At the time, I had just published my book *Play the Game Right: The Biography of Butch van Breda Kolf*, a pleasing documentary of the popular collegiate and professional basketball coach from 1951 to 1994. The speech was slated for seven-thirty in the evening, shortly after the conclusion of the all campus dinner.

Naturally, I adjusted my pill schedule accordingly, and when the dinner lingered on until close to nine o'clock, I became worried that my Parkinson's symptoms would soon show their ugly colors. I took an additional Sinemet pill just before the talk was about to begin. I rose to the occasion and gave the talk without any visible problems, but I felt less than "on" for the group. After I left the podium, I just didn't feel the speaker's high that normally accompanies the conclusion of an inspiring talk. After I had departed the affair, Ned Jesser explained to the Class of 1939 how my capabilities were impacted by the lateness of the hour. Jesser also is wedded to the clock. His wife Ruth suffers from Parkinson's.

For most of the first thirteen years I lived with Parkinson's, my social and business activities were not that affected by PD. At first, I seemed able to manage my pill rotation and superficially, at least, I was able to handle my job on Wall Street. I opted to become a "closet Parkinsonian," thinking I could conquer the disease by being tough. But gradually, my ability to write quickly and accurately deteriorated. I found myself memorizing trades because I couldn't write them down fast enough. Or I had to call a client back to verify the specifics of a trade. This fast-moving world of multimillion dollar transactions had no tolerance for tremors and freeze-ups. Conceptualizing swap ideas became more difficult. I calculated it would only be a matter of time before I was involved with a huge error. And so I retired. Gradually, the word of my Parkinson's factor became generally known. The handicapped stickers on both our family cars officially categorized us as such. When asked, we admitted the PD presence. (Note: The impact of PD on my business career is discussed in greater detail in Chapter 5A, "Attempts to Continue a Career.")

When I retired in 1999, I was fearful that the PD factor would make my days exceedingly long and boring. But one aspect of my personal background seemed unaffected by my Parkinson's disability. I had always been a very fast typist. For example, while serving on active duty just prior to the Cuban Missile Crisis of

1962, I was clocked at ninety-six words per minute at the U.S. Army Communications school in Ft. Gordon, Georgia. Furthermore, I loved to type and write. My skill had been reflected in my undergraduate leadership roles at Lafayette College in 1957 through 1960 when I was sports editor and then managing editor of the school's student newspaper. For the two years that immediately followed, I performed a similar function while pursuing my MBA at Wharton.[3] My ability to write material on a word processor seemed to motor on while my other basic actions were stalled by the PD factor. Although my typing speed slowed somewhat, and my number of errors increased, I still could type at a very fast pace and found, on occasion, that typing worked me out of some lingering off periods.

At first, I started writing about "things" in general. Then, I started to write about the Lafayette–Notre Dame basketball game played back in 1988. It was undoubtedly the greatest basketball victory in the school's history, as Lafayette romped over the Digger Phelps NCAA bound Irish by a score of 83–68.[4] Some 40 pages later the idea came to me: I should write the biography of the coach (i.e., Butch van Breda Kolff) who orchestrated the incredible Lafayette win over ND. In relatively short order, I had a retirement project and I was ready to roll!

---

[3]I was the editor-in-chief of the *Wharton Advocate,* which was published about every two or three weeks.
[4]Some would argue that Lafayette's only tournament win ever—a 72–71 win over ACC power Virginia University in the 1972 NIT was the school's greatest win ever. Dr. Tom Davis coached Lafayette at the time.

Finding a publisher for the book was virtually impossible. Although VBK was known among real basketball aficionados, he was not mainstream enough for the established publishing crowd to risk its capital on a rookie author such as myself. In my travels, I discovered the possibility of self-publishing the VBK book. Such a course would enable me to be the boss and I could write and/or publish at my own convenience. As I have learned, deadlines are not the best therapy for Parkinson's victims. When my wife yells at me to do something immediately, my first reaction is a fast tremble!

Upon visiting with Coach VBK, I discovered that he too suffered from Parkinson's. We bonded over this shared adversity, and we compared ailments and medications. Butch hated to take the appropriate pills and restricted himself to less than the full dosage. I, on the other hand, like to feel better, and so I frequently added on to my medication. I called such additional medication a bonus pill.

As the Parkinson's factor became more of an influence on my behavioral patterns, I continued to write and publish via my own publishing company, PAL Publishing Co. This book about PD is actually the fourth book I've written in the past five or six years.

In order to best survive the vicissitudes of PD, it is critical to have the elements of one's immediate environment well organized. Having a change of clothing and toilet articles neatly laid out in the morning is vital to getting a good start on the day. Having one's early morning medications ready is also important. More aspects of organizational matters are listed in a later chapter. Because so many of these activities are so basic, so mundane, it is easy for the PD victim to unintentionally ignore them, thus causing him even further frustration and delays in the morning.

Another means of mitigating the PD influence is exercise. I love golf and I have continued to play, albeit at reduced levels of coordination and resultant higher scores. Actually, when I first retired in 1999, I used the extra time available to practice my swing at the local driving range. Hitting golf balls at the range is vigorous exercise, in many cases more strenuous than playing eighteen holes!

One attribute of my golf game is that I don't hit the ball far enough to lose that many balls during a round. If you can elevate the ball so that it goes 150 yards straight at the target, you have a chance at breaking 100 at many golf courses. On the other hand, I dread hitting awkward shots (i.e., sand traps, severe downhill lies, etc) that require strong balance. In such cases, I frequently ask my playing partners for a "sympathy Mulligan," and I am able to move the ball without penalty.

On average, golf rounds take approximately four hours to complete. In my case, a full cycle of Parkinson's syndromes generally runs three hours. As I begin some golf games, I am off and may display rigid motor activity.

Once I take the appropriate dosage of pills, I turn on and my actions tend to resemble more "normal" human behavior. As the three-hour cycle approaches completion, I can feel my body heading for a short period of rigidity again. So when I play golf, a full behavioral cycle plus one hour of a second cycle may overlap my time on the links. The numbers are different depending on my starting time. Golf, or any human activity, becomes a process of adapting to the condition of the moment! Knowing where you are in your cycle and how long that cycle lasts may be more important than picking the right club!

You constantly hear golfers mention tempo as an intangible ingredient to a successful golf game. Your entire psyche gets into a zone, which allows you to cruise around the golf course as a virtual golfing machine. You function as if operating from the inside of a cocoon, which enables you to strip out all extraneous factors. With Mr. Parkinson at the controls, try as I may, it is so difficult to achieve this even tempo or golfer's zone.

The possibility of trapping yourself into an irrevocable position also adds to the problems of the PD victim. For example, I frequently take an afternoon nap, particularly after an evening of no sleep, in my mechanized lounger chair. Upon waking, I can push the switch and the chair literally launches me to a standing position. Recently, I was a bit overtired and slept in the chair for almost two hours, thus sleeping through one of the aforementioned three-hour pill units. When I woke up and tried to eject myself, the power switch wouldn't function. I suddenly realized that my wife, before departing for work, had turned off the light switch from another room. This was the same switch that controlled the electricity to the chair! I fortunately had enough thrust in my first foray to lift myself from the deep chair. As soon as possible, I scooted to my stable wheelchair. I had crossed over my pill time, so I was anxious to slip a cocktail of Sinemet, comtan, and mirapex before a further freeze-up took place.

Further complicating my days of late has been the redesign of our kitchen. By creating more space and an open-air quality, things are now further away from my reach. It will take time before I have the confidence to move around in this great room, and in the short term I have some challenges.

Another aspect of my PD has been my recent diet since my February 2004 appendectomy. The most revolutionary change has been no salt in my diet. For a guy who used to have three salt shakers on his desk, this has been quite a change. I have focused on more easily digestible foods, not eating too much meat. But recently I had one of my old favorites—quesadillas— at the Café Main in Madison. The highly seasoned cheese goodies tasted marvelous on the way down, but about half an hour after dinner, my salsa-seasoned meal was talking to me. Indigestion stayed with me until about five hours later. Although my hands functioned fairly well during this period, I had extreme difficulty mobilizing my legs and feet. It was like I was half on and half off.

With regard to meals, as just mentioned, I rarely order red meats anymore. I never know when I am going to have difficulty carving. One of my former life's favorite dishes was baked rigatoni with cheese as served by Poor Herbies restaurant in Madison. But most recently, I encountered a problem getting the dish into my mouth, as the noodles just wouldn't stay on the fork! My wife ordered a spoon from our waiter, and she wound up feeding me most of the dish. I was glad that the normally crowded restaurant was less than half full. Now, I tend to favor salmon and sea bass and items like the quesadillas, which are easy to manage. Only occasionally do I request outside help in feeding me my meal.

As much as possible, I have resisted becoming reliant on others to help me with routine chores. I feel the more independent I am, the better I will be able to handle the vice-like grip of PD. It is so easy to give in to the supportive members of one's family and social surroundings. The difficulties of climbing into and out of bed are quite familiar to most Parkinsonians. Often my wife has offered to help me extricate myself from under the covers. Here again, a plan of attack—a well-organized, repetitive method—serves the PD victim in good stead.

Nonetheless, being home alone is no fun, and I am fortunate to have a constant stream of friends who stop by and visit with me. Jokingly referred to as the Chatham Mens Club, the quartet of Doug Hobby, Ken Thompson, Kelly Dotson, and Raymond Monroe have spent tireless hours at my house and make my life considerably more tolerable. On occasion, Doug's son Brian stops by. Also, my Lafayette College classmate Alden Siegel has moved to the area and promises to become a regular participant in the Club's activities. (See photo.)

"The Basics

The victim of Parkinson's Disease usually has difficulty walking normally. *Walking,* assisted or unassisted, Parkinson style may involve a shuffle or short little steps rather than longer strides. When I arise in the middle of the night, I usually am in the off position, and so I drag my feet along the floor as I head for the bathroom. If I stop walking, sometimes it is difficult or im-

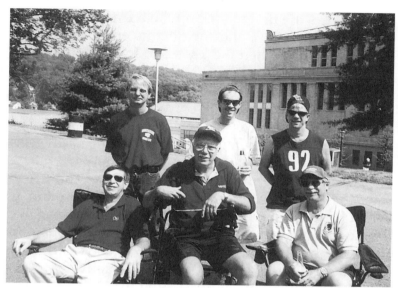

Members of the Chatham Mens Club are shown at a parking site before the Lafayette versus Marist football game in the fall of 2004. Front row sitting (left to right): Alden Siegel, Paul Luscombe, and Doug Hobby. Rear row standing: Kelly Dodson, Ken Thompson, and Raymond G. Monroe.
(Photo credit: Fran Nikles)

possible to get my feet moving again. Stopping to pivot into a sitting position can be very hard on my knees. If someone is with me, I have them "twist" me into the appropriate sitting position. Or sometimes, they move the chair to conform to my frozen position, and I just sit down. If I want to turn around, I frequently can accomplish a pivot by raising my right arm and using an elevated object, such as the top of the refrigerator or the towel hook on the back of the bathroom door.

My weak right side causes me havoc and probably is the culprit in most of the falls I have experienced. My right knee is the first to lock up. I have a brace, which I often forget to wear, and the doctors encourage me to exercise to strengthen the knee. Dr. John J. Knightly, a specialist in spinal surgery and general neurosurgery, performed a minimally invasive surgical procedure on my back that is supposed to correct my knee weakness, but more than a year has passed and my knee has shown no improvement. My right knee constantly feels like it is quite a bit heavier than its counterpart.

Depending on my activity for the day, I can use at least three means of getting from point A to point B. When I am playing golf, I prefer to use no support like a cane or a walker. Other than when restrictions preclude me from driving on the fairway, I usually only have to walk a few feet to the ball. I usually try to determine my club while approaching the ball. Using the roof of the cart as a prop, I can lift myself out of the cart and quickly snag the appropriate club and move into position to advance the golf ball. At recent golf outings, I have set out for the course without any prop, but eventually end up using my golf club as a cane when operating around the green. Rock Spring Country Club in West Orange had several elevated greens and a set of steps to climb in order to reach the putting surface. I used my putter to make the trip up and down those stairs. Such stairs on golf courses rarely are accompanied by any supportive railing.

I did take a hard fall inside the pro shop at the Locust Valley Golf Club in Coopersberg, Pennsylvania. After completing a full eighteen-hole round, I failed to change out of my spikeless golf shoes. One of the little nubs on the shoe caught in the well-worn carpeting, and I was sent flying. It also seemed the warped floors of the pro shop tilted the aging structure and helped to throw me off balance. Six months later, the Locust Valley Club was sold to a real estate development firm.

One of the new pieces of equipment that helps me keep mobile is called a rollader. It is essentially is a four-wheeled walker with a seat. This smartly colored vehicle is very lightweight (approximately fourteen pounds) and easily collapses to fit in the trunk or onto the back seat of a car. Although I generally exhibit a negative attitude about shopping at the mall, the walker is handy on those rare occasions when I must buy some Christmas or birthday gifts at a fancy store like Saks or Brooks Brothers. It is taxing for me to stand for any length of time without support, and so when I must wait on a line to pay for a gift, the walker with the seat is quite useful indeed. The walker is likewise functional when I take longer walks. I also bring my rollader to restaurants. As it is so difficult for me to find "the right chair" at unfamiliar restaurants, I find it best to bring my own. Many restaurants only offer uncomfortable booths, and the rollader gives me the option of sitting outside the cramped structure. The four point wingspan of the walker can make it a little difficult to pack in the car. Be advised not to force the walker (which I have dubbed my "tricycle" or "chariot") into a tight section of your trunk. We actually might have snapped the metal support bar when attempting to cram the walker into the trunk of my car.

After my appendectomy, an agent for the State of New Jersey visited my home to check up on the work being done by the Home Service Nurses Association. The agent was quite upset with my use of golf clubs as cane substitutes. So I now use the cane when appropriate, although I try to go without any support when I can.

Part of the problem relates to my absent-mindedness! My cane is constantly "missing in action." I have left it at any number of odd places. Last year, while attending the Patriot League basketball play-offs, I left the cane at the victory party for Lafayette's win over Colgate at the Show-Case Arena in Upper Marlboro, Maryland. Eventually Fred Brown, from the alumni relations department, held my cane in escrow until I could return to campus later in the spring.

With respect to walking, I seem to place a lot of importance on the proper fit of my socks. In fact, I frequently perform better when I wear my Dr. Shoales sneakers without any socks. When sockless, I seem to be able to have a better feel for Mother Earth.

This is a difficult policy to practice in cold weather (or some highly air conditioned restaurants). Some of my friends have caught a glimpse of my feet during dining hours when I discreetly remove my shoes to put on my socks.

Eating represents another problem area for many victims of the PD phenomenon. Most PD patients seem to like food that can be picked up by hand. Sandwiches, hot dogs and hamburgers, shrimp cocktails, the aforementioned quesadillas, Buffalo wings, and pizza are all easily managed.

My favorite pasta dishes (spaghetti, rigatoni, and ziti) are a little more difficult to handle. In the case of the pasta noodle, it is sometimes easier to stab the slippery item with your fork than to trying to maintain an edible portion on a spoon.

Voice level can be affected by Parkinson's. PD victims are known to drop their voice level in the middle of conversations. Their fatigue is accentuated as they are asked to repeat their remarks. Actually, I frequently tend to increase my volume when I am off, perhaps out of pure frustration. I forgo all efforts at tact and diplomacy, focusing only on whatever relatively meager physical act I want to accomplish. On the other hand, if I am in the middle of a Type B freeze-up, I am apt to half-mumble my words and drop my voice so that my remarks become unintelligible. In times like this, I usually have to repeat multisyllable words. When trying to express a complex thought, I sometimes forget midway through a lengthy sentence the point I was trying to make! However, by and large, I try to remain up tempo.

I also tend to mumble when I get up in the middle of the night to go to the bathroom. If my wife or a friend is assisting me, they frequently ask me to repeat my sentence. For that matter though, who is intelligible when they first get up at three a.m.?

The balance of the book will relate my Parkinson's experiences in the hopes that my problems and attempts at solutions will help soften the symptoms of this disease for you. I make no pretensions of having any medical background. My college training included one science course (geology), which I almost failed! I always have had a tendency to become squeamish at the sight of blood. Once, I passed out as a 2nd Lieutenant in the New Jersey National Guard while leading my platoon to a routine blood donor clinic.

My approach to my own version of Parkinson's disease has been to rely on the proper combination of medications and pills to maximize my on periods. The other alternative would entail a form of brain surgery. Many PD victims have opted for this route, some with great success and others with more limited results. The thought of brain surgery just makes me very squeamish.

Just a few general comments. I have always resisted being classified as a single personality type. My original Bache sales manager, Chris Sweeney, called me an enigma. My Lafayette College faculty advisor, George Strodach, said I was a modern stoic with some Epicurean characteristics. The Epicureans supposedly supported the theory of eat, drink, and be merry, for tomorrow you may die! I must admit I held a rather cavalier attitude toward handicapped people and the elderly. In my mind, I couldn't imagine how older people could enjoy themselves once they were beyond their physical and mental peak. Lacking any firm religious beliefs, I harbored the thought that no one checks out of this life alive, and I saw little value in postponing the inevitable.

I used to say that when I became a burden on society, someone should take me out and shoot me, rather than letting me drain society of its limited resources. When my own father died at the age of seventy-three, I was proud of his achievements in the banking world, but I was happy for his sake that he would suffer no longer while trying to fight the cancer wreaking havoc on his body. Now I wish he had lived a lot longer, which might have been possible if he had access to some of the products of modern cancer research. My mother's bout with Alzheimer's was a strain on my sister as Mom lingered on until she was eighty-five.

As a philosophy major in college, I was impressed by some of the tough theories of Nietzsche and Plato. Now that I am sixty-six years old and stricken with PD, I would have to say I favor a philosophic viewpoint whereby I am allowed to live my life to the fullest potential. I want to do my best to maximize the satisfaction of my on periods to the hilt! Outlining these thoughts will hopefully be useful to you all in doing the same.

Note: Parts of this chapter were paraphrased from author's earlier book entitled *Give Dad a Mulligan*, primarily the short story entitled "Play Golf with a Winning Handicap."

But not all pills are created equal. Every day is new and different, and not necessarily better.

Chapter 2A

Organizational Factors

Like many households in the twenty-first century, we maintain two or more phone lines for private use. With no teenage children left at home, my wife and I each maintain a separate line. Sometimes, visitors are surprised when I fail to answer my wife's telephone and just let the calling party leave a message on the internal system. When quizzed as to why I don't answer the phone, I explain that I am letting the phone take an accurate and thorough message from the caller. If I am in a partial freeze-up, I will be unable to take down any detailed notes. Also, the slightest hesitancy may slow down my writing capability. Even worse, I might forget to give my wife the message altogether! Furthermore, many of her calls are from telemarketers. It seems every time I answer her phone, my wife has just won a four-day trip to Orlando.

Forgetfulness and disorientation are among the common traits of Parkinson's victims. Flying by the seat of your pants is an admirable quality, indeed. But for the person stricken with PD, preparation and organization are vital not only for reacting to life's constantly changing environment, but for facing life's routine necessities as well.

The most critical schedule entails the timing of the patient's pill consumption. For my own method, I carry a small 4.5-inch long by 1-inch wide plastic pill box. They can be purchased at most pharmacies or at suppliers of equipment for the elderly. Some prefer a larger size than the one I use. The container is segmented into the seven days of the week, with each of the days marked with a capital letter. The lettering is bold and sits on a blue base. As you view the box from the top, it reads "S—M—T—W—T—F—S"

In my own mind, I substitute the days of the week for one twenty-four-hour period with each letter signifying a specific three-hour unit of any given day. Obviously, $7 \times 3 = 21$, and I use the second "S" chamber to house capsules that I might use in the middle of the night. In essence, the letters stand for the following pill compositions (which I jokingly refer to as "cocktails"):

Time of Day	Letter	Pills Taken
6 a.m.	S	2 carbidopa (25mg/100mg)
		1 mirapex (1.0 mg)
		1 comtan (200mg)
9 a.m.	M	2 corbi, 1 Comtan
12 noon	T	2 corbi, 1 Comtan,
		1 mirapex, 1 Proscar (prostate related)
3 p.m.	W	2 corbi, 1 Comtan
6 p.m.	T	2 corbi, 1 Comtan, 1 Mirapex
9 p.m.	F	2 corbi, 1 Comtan
Midnight	S	1 Sinemet CR (25/100 mg),
		2 Flomax (prostate related)

Note: All strengths of pills shown for "Sunday" apply throughout the "menu." Figures in parentheses indicate dosage.

"Be careful not to lose your pills" is probably a very obvious piece of advice. However, many pockets may not be the most secure location in which to carry your lifeline. Some pockets are too shallow and the pills may slip out when you are seated at a particular angle. I find myself constantly tapping my left pocket to see that my pills are properly stored. On occasion, I have had to retrace my steps and have found the pillbox in the crease of a chair I had been sitting in.

The two units located at the ends of the pillbox (which my friends and I label the "book ends") are often taken in almost total darkness. The strategic location of each chamber more or less ensures that I am taking the right dosage at the right time. I like to take my pills with Dannon natural spring water, because I find that twisting the cap back on the plastic bottle less trouble than reclosing Evian bottles. I would leave the cap loosened, but I am afraid that in the night I might knock the bottle over and mar some woodwork in the area. My urologist also has me taking two medications to control my prostate. These drugs have been critical in bringing down my PSA from 4.2 to 1.2 over a period of time. I have integrated these drugs into my Parkinson's schedule for consistency purposes.

I try to totally refill the box between noon and three p.m. every day. I try to note which pills are running low and to call the local pharmacist when I am down to a one- or two-day supply. Sometimes, the pharmacist may have to call the doctor for permission to refill my prescriptions, and this takes a little extra time. If I have waited until no pills are left in my inventory, and if I am also delayed by the doctor, the pharmacist will usually advance me a few extra pills until he gets the word from the doc. Due to the weakness of my right side, I try to carry the pill box in my left-hand pants pocket at all times. If I am wearing a sports jacket or a sports shirt with an upper left pocket, I may tuck the pillbox there, but still on the left side. The pillboxes that contain the refills are stored collectively in a plastic Hefty bag with a one-zip feature. The Hefty bag is left on the top of my desk in a prominent location. Other than when I am off premises, my plastic pill bag never leaves the house. It literally is my lifeline.

Before retiring every night, I try to make sure my pills are located in their usual parking spot on the end table next to my bed. They are protected on the near side by the remote for the TV and on the far side by the intercom button I use to ring my wife in times of distress. Only one water bottle is required to get me through the night. I try to limit what goes on the top of this little table, but invariably other unauthorized items invade the sacred territory.

At night, taking pills is a bit tricky. A modicum of light is provided by the closet light, which—when lit— seeps through the slits of the louver doors. I find that knowing my pillbox will be at the same station properly facing me so that the letters are right-side up enables me to take the medicine without getting out of bed. Isolating the single Sinemet CR has helped me consume that pill at its appointed hour, which (until an important recent change) was between four and five in the morning.

One morning recently, I actually dreamed that I had taken my jump start opening salvo of four pills. While I lay asleep dreaming, comfortably assuming that my pills were working for me, they in fact were sitting in my pillbox and time was working against me. The longer I waited to take the pills, the longer it would take for them to kick in and take their salutary effect. When I finally did awake and began to wonder why my meds had not influenced my body's activities, I checked the pillbox and saw the full chamber for the six a.m. feeding.

Generally speaking, it takes roughly twenty to thirty minutes for the opening salvo to impact my nervous system. After taking these four pills, I can sit on the edge of the bed, motionless, perhaps frozen, while waiting for the pills to have their desired effect. Then, wham! A surge of energy jolts my body, my feet start to twist and turn, and soon I am jumping off into space. For the Parkinsonian, this rush of motion is probably the best feeling in the world! If I have an important obligation that morning and want to start the day, I often doubt that the pills will do their job. So far, my fears have been unfounded, as I don't recall a void on the part of the six a.m. dosage.

Sometimes I fail to organize my next morning's garb because I had difficulty getting to bed the night before. My efforts to get dressed are impaired as I have probably wildly thrown my clothes onto my organizer chair that sits near my bed. Such disarray usually results in my wearing the same clothes as I did the day before. I vow to neaten up the chair during my shower time (between eight and nine a.m.) if I am on.

One staple that I keep near the bed is a walker without the wheels. This fairly stationary gadget helps me stand up when I first get out of bed and may be used to store some of my critical clothing for the next morning. As I get dressed in the early a.m., this walker helps me maneuver my feet or hands throughout the dressing process.

The following items frequently typify my early morning wardrobe:

- *Shoes or sneakers with Velcro straps rather than shoelaces.* For me, these slide on fairly easily. I put on socks later in the morning.
- *Warm-up pants or shorts with elastic waists.* I find it somewhat critical to put my right foot and leg into the pants before my left. I drape the elastic part of the pants over my right knee, and thereby create some pressure to help in elevating the left pants leg. It is essential that these pants have pockets to carry my pill supply. The pants process can take a long time, and my wife frequently helps me get my shorts or slacks into position. This is an immense help to my demeanor and to my schedule.
- *FTL (Fruit of the Loom) underwear* seems the easiest to pull up, and this is especially important after going to the bathroom in the middle of the night, a time when it is sometimes difficult to obtain balance. FTL underwear may, however, produce some friction when I first try to pull up my warm-up pants or shorts. If I remain patient, the pants eventually inch their way into the proper position.
- *Lightweight, baggy sweatshirt or vest sweater.* After getting my arms and neck through the appropriate apertures, the most difficult aspect of donning the pullover is just that, pulling the lower hem of the item down to my waistline. Eventually, gravity prevails and soon I am ready to roll.

Another organizational aspect of coping with PD involves planning one's routes around the house (or for the traveler, around the hotel room). When at home, once I am dressed, I descend the stairs to our living room. I leave my wheelchair in a strategic location, facing the kitchen door and in the locked position. From the living room, I push the wheelchair into the kitchen, and I spin the chair so that it backs into the stove. I then use the top of the refrigerator for leverage and sit down and get ready for breakfast.

My wife, a perfectionist about preparing meals, has everything organized for me! Juice in the fridge, coffee grounds in the percolator, scrambled egg and bacon in the pan on the stove ready to be cooked, and enough fresh fruit and pastry to feed the Ukrainian Army.

Traveling overnight or for a vacation requires a special organizational effort. Most critically, I must make sure that my pill supply sufficiently covers the length of time I will be away. The schedule I outlined earlier lists a grand total of twenty-four pills. I consume twelve carbidopa and levodopa tablets per day, and I obviously use these up the most quickly. I store toilet articles in a separate kit because they generate so much moisture.

Traveling light is indeed a virtue. I try to make an estimate of the climate I will be visiting and to not bring a wardrobe for every conceivable weather condition. If I am wrong, I try to tough it out or layer for a day or so. A more serious problem arose on a particular vacation when I realized that I had put on a lot of weight since my previous vacation. Most obviously affected was my mid-section, where I ballooned from a 35W to a 40W, adding thirty-five pounds to my overall weight. By sitting around and eating too much, I have altered my physique to resemble the shape of my desk chair. I definitely need to get on an exercise program. For our Florida trip in April of 2004, I tried on all my Bermuda shorts and swimming trunks before packing. To look for specific sizes just before catching the cab to the airport puts too much stress on the traveling. Items with elasticized waists seemed to look the best on me. When I look in the mirror, all I can think is "Pear-Shape Paul."

Upon arriving at a travel destination, I take a few minutes to organize a route to the bathroom from the bed. I may line up some straight back chairs, if available, as a means of support in walking to my objective. Open space creates ambiguity in my mind, and this leads to my standing still for a few seconds. In those few seconds, my body can become as frozen as a block of ice.

If possible, I also try to lie on the same side of the bed as I do when at home. If the motel provides a clock, I move it to my side of the bed so that I can time my mid-evening pills.

Among my Parkinson's issues is the fact that I forget to write down appointments. Prior to developing this trait, I used to keep a very meticulous appointment book. However, living the casual life of a retiree, I find I rarely wear a suit jacket or sports jacket any more, and have no spare pockets to carry a modest size booklet. Every day seems the same! There is nothing special about a Friday versus a Saturday. Even if I do carry the appointment book, I frequently miss the announcement or am frozen and can't write anything down. As a partial replacement, I bought a box calendar featuring two-inch write-in spaces for each day. This sits right in front of me at my computer and is a constant reminder that I should be thinking of my schedule for the week, the month, and perhaps further into the year. If I am having trouble writing, I try to type a little sticker for the calendar. For medical appointments, I have the doctor's office write me up a card and I staple it to the calendar. If any forward time is involved, I also ask the aide to call me a day or two ahead of time.

In case you were wondering just how my handwriting appeared, I have jotted a short message below for your inspection:

Sometimes, a message that appears perfectly clear to me on the day it was written can be totally incomprehensible twenty-four hours later. I have a particular problem trying to decipher numbers that I have written. It could be sevens and ones, or fives and zeros. Regardless, I tend to get them mixed up!

When I receive notices of meetings or outings that I want to attend, I not only mark my calendar but I also save the descriptive flier in my address book. Football and basketball schedules, particularly the New York

Jets and Lafayette College, are pasted in the address book as soon as they are announced.

Forgetting where you put your car keys, your wallet, your glasses, can be a source of panic for the PD victim (and for that matter, anyone without PD!). I call the drawer on the right side of my antique computer desk my magic drawer, and whenever someone borrows any important item, I tell them to return the same to my magic drawer. When I retire at night, I try to unload my pockets and place the items in this spot. As much as possible, I store my address book and key household bills in the same location. Right now, the magic drawer is bulging at the seams!

Similarly, I try to organize the miscellaneous equipment relating to my golf game. Certain little additional items have helped me improve my game. For example, very long tees seem to help me elevate the ball off the ground when I am using my oversized driver. I must purchase these tees at the East Orange Golf Club. Yes, they are legal. When most other golfers use them, a pop-fly is generally the result. Also, I play in my prescription sunglasses, which I always have handy when I am organizing my gear for golf. Bifocal or trifocal eyeglasses are troublesome when trying to get down to the ball. Without my distance sunglasses, I tend to top the ball, because the ordinary reading glasses bring the ball closer to me than it really is!

A glove is not necessary, but it helps. At this point in time, only one pair of shoes fits my feet![1] So all this pe-

---

[1]Since my brace won't fit into my normal golf shoes, I purchased a pair of size 14 sneaker-golf shoes. I wear my regular shoe on my left foot and the new size 14 shoe and my brace on the other foot.

ripheral equipment goes in a shoe bag marked "ECCC" (i.e., the logo for Essex County Country Club), which I received as a favor for playing in the Seniors Tourney there a few years ago. In my pre-Parkinson days, I was never so neat!

Not all pills are created equal. Every day is new and different, and not necessarily better. It is most difficult to predict how the Sinemet CR pill will influence my morning routine. Some mornings, the CR kicks in in less than an hour, sometimes it does its best work after an hour and a half. Recently, when I had a cold in Florida, it seemed the CR didn't kick in at all! After such a build-up, a void! Also, one morning when the CR did kick in, I rushed to put on my warm-up pants and on my way downstairs, I realized I had put the pants on backwards! Once I was on, I switched the warm-up pants to their proper position. I have also been known to put both legs in the same pants leg.

Action on the stairs can be treacherous, but I find that the thirteen steps leading to our second floor can be somewhat therapeutic. To date, walking down the stairs early in the morning or climbing the stairs at night seems to get my motor going. One morning, however, I was for-tunate to catch myself before advancing too far. Inad-vertently, I had put on a pair of warm-up pants without any side pockets. To carry my pills, I needed a pocket, so I hastily selected a dressy shirt which I left unbuttoned. As I started my descent, I felt the tail of this shirt grab the banister. Fortunately, I was not moving in one of my "let's get this over as soon as possible" moods, and I was able to stop on the stair and untangle the shirt.

Being **off** is just the worst. At the extreme, nothing moves. I sit in a chair or on the edge of the bed, and I am temporarily paralyzed. No matter how hard I try to will myself back to the on position, more often than not I am just locked in until time passes and the most recent dose of PD medicine goes to work. It is so frustrating to have so much to do and then be unable to do anything! I may be locked in sitting at the computer and be unable to turn it on or operate the mouse. Even with two hands on the mouse!

I grow very impatient waiting for this rigidity to pass. Therefore, I grunt and groan, whirl my arms in the air, and as a last resort, call for help from my wife or whoever might be visiting me. The need to go to the bathroom seems to aggravate the anxiety of the off position. I retain my own version of a porta-john (i.e., an empty Gatorade bottle) in the living room just in case I have an emergency.

Once back on, I try to capitalize on the on time as best I can. I used to be able to make it through an entire round of golf without going off, at least to the extent listed above. But as my PD has degenerated, I find I have more difficulty accomplishing this feat. Either I have to sit out a hole or two, possibly accept some sympathy Mulligans, or I must cheat a little bit. If I am unable to hit the t-shot at least 100 yards, I may walk the ball out to the 100 yard mark and play the hole from there. For score purposes, I take nothing better than an eight on such holes.

I am not on the course to win any prizes. I am out there for the exercise and the friendship. Perhaps we all should be on the course with the same idea!

Better yet, I even get to drive the golf cart! This turns out to be quite a privilege for me now that I am can't drive a car. I do find that I press my right foot a little hard on the accelerator. Plus I did accidentally bump my opponent's cart the other day when we were in close quarters on the tee. So far, I have yet to fall asleep while driving the cart. I have, however, dozed while waiting to hit behind a slow moving foursome.

Some golf courses restrict the use of carts to cart paths only, and this puts a lot of strain on my playing ability. Many of my partners let me hit my shot from near the cart path, simply moving the ball over the fairway to be equidistant from the hole. It's not tournament golf, but it's fun and I get to drive the cart!

The more difficult courses are laden with elevated greens and tees, sand traps that are over one's head, and a whole host of challenging obstacles. When invited to these courses, I usually decline because of the problems I have climbing and descending the hills. To preserve the essentially beautiful examples of nature, management of these courses does not allow the golf cart to go within thirty to forty yards of the obstacle. Unfortunately, this can really wear me down.

Recently, my most frequent golfing partner Doug Hobby observed that my long putts were more accurate than my shorter ones. I thought about this comment and then I realized the reason. My body tends to cramp up or experience stress when I stand for a long time. My first putt is obviously en route shortly after I reach the green. My second or third putt is usually several minutes later, and should be in the sequence of which golfer is further from the hole. As golf's protocol takes over, the pain of waiting intensifies and I tend to rush my shorter putts; not a lot, but just enough to miss. Golf is a game of inches.

On rainy days when golf is not a favorable option, I frequently work on my Class of 1960 article for the Lafayette College *Alumni News*. I must write at least three articles a year for this publication, and generating news about retired sixty-five year olds is not always so easy. On a rainy Memorial Day weekend, I recently decided to create some news by setting up the Class of 1960 golf tournament. As the response grew stronger and stronger, my self-esteem grew as well. I started to really feel good about myself. Almost everyone I called accepted the invitation. In no time, I had a course to play, a time and a date, and sixteen players ready to participate. I would ask some celebrities later in the week, some alumni who have been inducted into Lafayette's athletic Hall of Fame and who also play golf. Maybe we could even include a women's foursome or two. As I grew more and more excited about the possibilities of the tourney, my dyskinesia started to amplify and soon I hit the disconnect button while talking on the phone with at least two potential players. The same phenomenon took place when I really got into marketing ideas. As I got excited, my whole body started to move around and it is hard to keep from hitting the wrong button on the phone. I also knocked over a whole box of peanuts, which I struck with the back of my chair.

Being a holiday, I couldn't obtain any support such as updated phone numbers from the Lafayette Alumni Relations Department. I did, however, leave a message with Joe Samaritano, alerting him to my tournament activities (i.e., times, date, location, etc.) and my hope that his department could send out an information postcard to the Class of 1960. While I had the momentum and the positive energy, I wanted to accomplish as much as I could. I was definitely on and could hardly wait for the next day to arrive. I just hoped my "busy hands" wouldn't disconnect any more classmates!

The group golf tournament routine has become a bit commonplace of late. Everyone's doing it! I am glad I was proactive and telephoned the people I did. As the summer schedule unfolded, as my mail flowed in, many such contrived tournaments threatened to dilute my little gathering. I was hoping that my event had some allure for retirees because it would take place on a Tuesday (most others were Friday), before lunch, and at a course of modest difficulty and length, but attractive and interesting nonetheless. The cost of fifty-five dollars was also quite competitive!

Subsequently, as my mood shifted, I worried I had created an event that I couldn't handle. But my pal Hobby was helping me out and my second guessing soon disappeared. I just hoped my PD would cooperate the day of the outing!

Generalizing about the nature of one's Parkinson's experiences is very difficult. Every day is different. One day, you feel like walking the golf course, the next day you don't care if you ever play again. I consider myself to be somewhat emotionally stable, but it is amazing the extent to which I react differently on one day to the same stimuli I faced the day before. If you detect some contradictions in this text, it is not because of any untruths. Sometimes, when comparing behavior on a week-to-week or month-to-month basis, it doesn't even seem like I'm the same person!

Looking back, I am amazed in some cases that I could accomplish what I did. In others, I wonder what kept me from finishing a project.

Chapter 2B

Financial Management and the Costs Relating to a Parkinson's Drug Program

My father was not a big believer in the effectiveness of insurance policies. He constructed his own insurance pool, and gradually built a financial safety net consisting mostly of common stocks. The core of the portfolio consisted of common stock from Peoples Bank, for which he worked most of his career. His holdings essentially made him the second largest owner of the bank. In his waning days, he continually admonished me not to sell the Peoples Bank common.[1] The portion of his portfolio relating to Peoples Bank stock was "passive" in nature, and only functioned when stock became available in the marketplace. From this standpoint, he was a classic example of the "buy and hold" or, more precisely, the "buy and accumulate" philosophy of investing.

---

[1]The Peoples Bank, officially named the Peoples National Bank & Trust Company of Belleville, New Jersey, was a very tightly held bank with fewer than a hundred shareholders. In the mid 1980s, the Peoples was acquired by the Valley National Bank, primarily a New Jersey banking concern.

The second portion of my father's nest egg was a financial juggernaut! Similar to a miniature hedge fund, he flipped in and out of new issues of common stock. He used a variety of Wall Street sources, the most active of which was the charismatic Tom Jones of Hornblower & Weeks. He boasted that a single trade with Hornblower covered my spring tuition fee at Wharton Graduate School in 1962.

Portfolio performance was not compared with the Dow Jones Index or any other measure. By using his own program, he could cover the costs of my sister's and my college education, afford a new Cadillac every two years, and have the option to seek the best medical assistance in the event of potential family health crises. He died in 1973 before the medical advances in dealing with prostate cancer had become widely known. Prior to discovering his prostate problem, he seemed more preoccupied with treating his menier's disease, an affliction of the inner ear, which made him very dizzy and prone to fainting. I remember driving him to Hackensack General Hospital (in New Jersey), where he would get himself checked by a top specialist in inner ear problems. Regardless, I don't sense that he lacked the funds to pay for the best medical care when the prostate cancer struck his body. I suspect, like many men of that era, he failed to recognize the cancer's symptoms until after the disease had spread beyond any known cure.

After his passing, my mother was fortunate that he had set up a financial plan using the trust department of the First Bank & Trust of Boynton Beach, Florida. The point man for the program was twenty-nine-year-old Jeff Keating. He later left the bank and started his own investment advising firm and he continued to monitor my mother's program until she died in 1985. My sister and I still maintain modest investment accounts managed by Keating.[2]

Following my father's constant advice, I embarked on a savings plan that not only included a significant ownership interest in the common stock of my employer(s) but also diversified into what I perceived to be attractive investments.[3] Oddly enough, some of my best performers were from the New Jersey banking sector. I traded the portfolio, when appropriate, but over the years the SEC and other regulators limited the potential appreciation in comparison to the era when my father was active. I also followed my father's recommendation of maintaining a low level of personal debt. Unfortunately, he offered little advice on how to structure a health insurance plan.

I was thirty-five when my father died. I was in good shape, played a lot of golf and basketball, and contracting Parkinson's disease was something I thought I might experience, if at all, when I turned eighty or so. Also, during most of my thirty-seven-year career, health insurance was provided by my employer and in fact endured a year and a half beyond my retirement. In my mind, there was no need to allocate funds to help pay for PD, which wouldn't impact my health until close to the end of my life expectancy.

When I did actually retire and the grace period of Morgan Stanley coverage had run out, I enlisted the

---

[2]Jeff Keating details the U.S. economy during the high rate period of the 1980s in the foreword he wrote for my book *Howard Powerless*.
[3]The best employee stock investment plan was that of Morgan Stanley (and previously Dean Witter), in which the company specified matching programs during good years in the cycle.

help of Sal Petruzzellis, a LC graduate and basketball buddy of mine, who helped me set up a health insurance program for my wife and me. After a thorough search, I signed up for a UnitedHealthcare health insurance plan. In my case, because of the known Parkinson's disease factor, it was difficult to find *any* health insurer to take me on. By default, I accepted the UHC program.

The costs associated with my particular Parkinson's disease drug program are outlined in Exhibit 1.

Costs of Parkinson's-Related Drugs
(as of January 1, 2005)

Name of Drug	Pills/month	Cost/month
Carbidopa/Levodopa (12); 25/100 (brand name: Sinemet)	360	$173.32
Comtan (6); 200 mg	180	460.78
Sinemet CR (1); 25/100	30	33.82
Mirapex (3); 1mg	90	225.89
TOTALS	660	$888.51

Notes:
Figure inside parentheses equals daily intake.
Cost at CVS Pharmacy, 471 Main St., Chatham, NJ.
In my case, I have been denied insurance coverage for these drugs because of pre-existing conditions or earnings tests. My principal relief comes in the form of a medical tax deduction on my federal returns.

For three years, I paid fairly steep insurance premiums to the UnitedHealthcare, as I maintained a joint policy for my wife and myself. The most glaring oversight became apparent when my wife broke her arm at the Lago Mar resort in Ft. Lauderdale, Florida. UHC claimed there was a lapse in my coverage at the time. I ended up paying for my wife's medical fees associated with her arm (slightly less than $900) plus any other significant health expenses from my own portfolio of stocks and bonds.

When I turned sixty-five in 2003, I became eligible for Medicare under the auspices of the Social Security Administration. The Bankers National Life of Iowa stepped in and has become my secondary source of medical coverage. Despite my conscientious efforts to effectuate this transition, UHC claimed there was a lapse in coverage from a joint policy to one strictly for coverage of any of my wife's emergencies.

Still, a huge void exists in my health insurance coverage as far as prescription drugs are concerned. I have received notices of companies offering programs for coverage, but upon further examination, the time span that I have lived with PD or my level of taxable income have acted as reasons for the insurance companies to reject my application.

And so, I am left to take my prescription costs as an itemized deduction on my federal income tax return. Under existing law, the amount of these expenses combined with all my other medical expenses, must exceed 7.50 percent of my total income. If my income for a given year is $100,000, then my total medical expenses would have to exceed $7,500 before I could take an itemized deduction for medical costs. For example, using the numbers shown in Figure 1, my federal tax deduction for the given year would be $3,162.12.

Figure 1

Annual Income = $100,000
$\times$ 7.50% = $7,500 (minimum medical expense base)
Amount of prescription drug expenses incurred = $10,662.12
Amount of prescription drugs taken as deduction = $3,162.12

If I calculate my deduction using prescriptions as a part of my 7.5 percent base, then all other medical deductions would be allowable in full.

One of the more bizarre scenarios related to the bills associated with Parkinson's disease (and other illnesses as well) is the practice of consumers in the United States purchasing their drugs through Canadian pharmacies. The price disparity can be absurdly wide, and continues to exist despite a universal cry to narrow the gap. The most expensive of the drugs is Comtan, which costs about 33 percent more at the Chatham, New Jersey CVS (see Exhibit 1) than at the British Columbia pharmacy located more than three thousand miles away. Novartis, located about five miles from me in East Hanover, New Jersey, manufactures Comtan.

A July 12, 2005 *Wall Street Journal* article entitled "Parkinson's Drug May Trigger Compulsions" by Scott Hensley article asserts that, according to findings at the Mayo Clinic, some users of mirapex have exhibited extensive tendencies toward heavy gambling. Also mentioned was a tendency toward sexual fixations (i.e., "pornography") and carrying on extra-marital affairs. "The Mayo Clinic doctors think Mirapex . . . may be hyper-stimulating for some people and send their search for pleasure into overdrive," Hensley writes. Physicians are grappling with the problem and trying to discern the extent of the side-effects listed. Stay tuned!

Perhaps the most depressing part of Parkinson's disease is the matter of being unable to drive a car. Driving is not allowed because I can fall asleep at any time without any advance warning.

Chapter 3

Analysis of Sleep Phenomenon

Sleep should be a very pleasant topic. A chance to relax your body and rest your mind, sleep is a vital part of our daily routine and key to the rest of our physical performance during the day. But in today's competitive environment, professional businesspeople tend to opt for some advantage by getting to work a little bit earlier and/or working later. The work climate at many firms has shifted from a comfortable nine-to-five regimen to a twenty-four/seven pattern—business can be conducted twenty-four hours a day, seven days per week. Also, in a service-oriented economy such as we have in the United States, many take multiple jobs or jobs requiring irregular hours. Sleep becomes a haphazard, when available privilege. Prior to my retirement in 1999, I too was swept into this competitive mode and found myself rising at four-thirty a.m. to do my sit-ups and watch the early news before cleaning up and catching the 6:09 a.m. train to New York City. Almost until the day I retired in July 1999, I felt I just had to get into my office on the sixtieth floor of World Trade Center #2 by seven-fifteen a.m.

Few if any of my clients were in at this early hour, but certain meetings were taking place and it was helpful to get my calls lined up and just generally organize myself. Because of the lack of telephone interference, I also was able to write some market letters and daily comments at this early hour. Perhaps some of my current problems with sleep stem from this competitive syndrome. When I retired, I found it difficult to sleep past five in the morning, and on many occasions I was up early working on my word processor.

From the Parkinson's viewpoint, perhaps the main problem I have with sleeping originates with the way I wake up. Usually, I go to bed between ten and eleven at night, and I sleep solidly for ninety minutes to two hours. When I am aroused from this sound sleep, I find myself to be totally frozen. At first, all I can do is blink my eyelids. The paralysis is overwhelming and very frightening. My first thoughts are: How am I going to get out of this bed and into the bathroom? Will my legs be nimble enough so they don't buckle, resulting in an injurious fall?

The key is to start moving any body part, however slightly, that responds to my brain's command. Usually, my left side is the most reliable, and so I stretch out my left hand—a process which may take several minutes—and try to lock onto a portion of the headboard. Suddenly, my left knee swings into action. My right side seems to get some feeling and starts to inch along. Although I am in the off position, the minimal body movements help me straighten up so that I can get out of the bed and head toward the bathroom. If I am unable to straighten myself up, I make a wide swooping motion with my right arm and land it in a fist-like position so that I can leverage myself up into a vertical position. If the time is five-forty in the morning or so, this also puts me in an efficient position to take my opening morning pills.

When I originally encountered this need to break out of a deep sleep because of my own paralysis, I thought the process took approximately fifteen to twenty minutes. But recently, I have timed this maneuver, and find that it takes just two to three minutes from the time I start to unravel my body from a sleeping or crouched position to a stance where my back is straight in the air and both feet are on the ground. At times earlier than five o'clock, I am off to the bathroom with the intention of returning to the bedroom unescorted by my wife. If the time is approximately five-forty-five a.m., I ring my wife on the intercom and she helps me get dressed in a matter of minutes. I am ready to roll and challenge our stairs to the living room as soon my meds become effective. This generally occurs when my feet start to feel active and suddenly I am up responding to the surge generated by the early morning pills. Once on the stairs, I feel the medicine take a firmer hold as my feet generate more feeling. A cardinal rule is that, once on the stairs, I must keep moving.

Prior to my official morning wake-up activity, I am usually roused out of bed by the urge to go to the bathroom. These round trips usually occur around midnight, two a.m. and four a.m. Depending on the time, upon returning to the bedroom, I take a modest dose of my medicines. Between midnight to one a.m., I take

one carbidopa and lopadopa (a.k.a. Sinemet) along
with one flomax (prostate related). As I get into bed, I
try to plan my next move out of bed! I want my knees
to be facing in the "exit" direction. And so I get into
bed, pushing myself as far to the right as I can so that I
can roll back to that favorable position. Invariably, my
right leg gets caught in the sheet, or my skull backs
right onto the headboard. Often, I am just too close to
the edge of the bed. I use some of the moves taught me
by the physical therapists in Livingston (Christopher
and Jonathan) to fine-tune my location. I sometimes
tune in the TV to help me center myself and to relax my
mind a little bit. Once properly aligned, and once the
TV is turned off, I tend to fall soundly asleep for another two hours, possibly a little longer. Again, when I
awaken between three and four a.m., I am frozen but
usually not as solidly as at one o'clock. And the journey
back and forth from the bathroom is repeated. A little
more stress and strain, another dabble with the TV, and
I am usually set for another interlude of sleep.[1]

Enter the power pill, Sinemet CR (stands for "controlled release"). This pill can, at times, have an amazing impact on me. Approximately seventy-five to ninety
minutes after taking one of these little devils, I sometimes feel I am in the maximum on position, but only for
a very short period, possibly five to eight minutes. I feel
like I could play full court basketball on the spot!

For the longest time, I tried to time the Sinemet CR
pill so that its favorable impact coincided with the ap-

---

[1]Also, I have this innate fear of lost circulation in my legs and I
may want to get up just to give them a little stimulation.

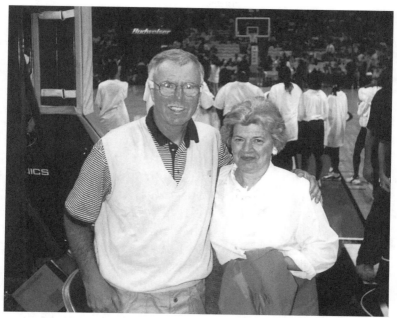

Author Luscombe and his wife Cinnie enjoy going to sporting events together, shown here at a Miami Heat home basketball game in 2001. (Photo credit: Miami Heat basketball fan)

proximate time I wanted to get up and get dressed. Without such a power nudge, it sometimes took me forever (almost an hour) to get my clothes and shoes on. Therefore, I liked to be awake about four-fifteen a.m. so that I could take the Sinemet CR and have it kick in a little before six in the morning. That is when I take my major dose of medicine for the day (i.e., two carbidopa levadobas, one mirapex, and one comtan). Usually, if this chain of events worked out, I was dressed and out of bed and headed downstairs between the Sinemet CR influence and when I took this morning cocktail. For a while, I thought I had beaten the system!

Over the past few years, I've found that I tend to sleep in two-hour increments (or slightly less). Although I dose off unexpectedly during the day, by and large I have eliminated the nap that was such an integral part of my life up to just a few years ago. I find that if I lie down and nap, it takes me forever to get my psyche up and running for the day.

While looking like a sound strategy on paper, sometimes this CR maneuver is just difficult to time. Perhaps all pills are not created equal! On a number of occasions, I took my CR pill at four-fifteen a.m. and awaited favorable developments by five-forty-five a.m. In the absence of any stimulus, I then took my regular morning cocktail at five-forty-five a.m., and if the benefits of the CR did not materialize, I had to sit and wait another thirty minutes before the regular pills kicked in. Since I dressed early when I thought the CR was working, I literally was like a commuter from a remote location who must sit at the train station and wait for the next train to come in. It's no fun to sit rigid for half an hour in the early morning. On some mornings, I chanced the stairs. Other mornings, I chose to wait until the pills kicked in.

I have experimented slightly with the CR pill and the results were near disastrous. One pill per day is good enough for me! And actually, if I am really sound asleep, which is not that often, I have been known to sleep right through the benefits of the CR.

Upon hearing of my results with the CR pill, Dr. Waters suggested that I take the pill at bedtime rather than four a.m., and to possibly take one Sinemet in the middle of the night if I felt a degree of insomnia. I have had some luck with this practice and some sleep-through voids. Perhaps more experimentation is called for with the CR.

Sometimes, especially in the middle of the night, I have difficulty in extracting the pill(s) from their respective cartridge in my pillbox. This occurs when I awaken from a deep sleep, can hardly move, and am anxious to take a Sinemet CR or my jump start four-pill cocktail. Quite often I take the pill(s) while lying in the prone position and sliding some of the water into the side of my mouth. Usually, the transfer using this position works, although in April 2004, I missed my mouth with both the Sinemet CR and later on in the morning with the mirapex postioin of my daily opener.

When I felt the Sinemet CR drop out of my mouth, it fell very close to my chin and folded arms. In a series of very delicate moves, I probed the area around my chest. Gradually, as I lifted my head, I saw the vagrant pill and popped it into my mouth. About ninety minutes later, I sat up to take my four-pill dosage. This time the mirapex pill failed to negotiate the transfer, and rolled somewhere out of sight. Remaining calm and not wanting to wake up my wife, I reached the light next to my bedstead and searched the area around my feet. When I moved my shoes, I found the lone pill lying next to the bed post. I was able to grasp the pill between my left fingertips and bring it up to my mouth.

To facilitate swallowing my pills, I keep a bottle of Sprite or some bottled water at hand. One difficulty that seems to constantly reoccur is the opening and closing of one of these bottles. The activity seems to activate a tremor in my right hand, or leaves it entirely rigid. I hate to put the bottle back in place without the top securely tightened, in case I should knock it over while wrestling with the bed covers. With a little patience, though, I can secure the top.

Once downstairs in the morning, I turn on my computer and possibly have a cookie from a stack left near
my desk by my wife. During the day, I will undoubtedly fall asleep while working on the computer. I somehow rationalize that these little impromptu naps will
compensate for the less than seven hours of sleep that
I get in my actual bed.

In my case, I find that many factors can influence
the achievement of a favorable sleep. If I have had dinner at an unusually late hour, and then try to go to bed
right away, I may have trouble with indigestion. For
several weeks during 2003, my wife worked late hours
on Sunday nights, and we would have dinner afterward at the Café Main, which served dinner until ten
o'clock. We virtually had the restaurant to ourselves.
But after the delightful meal, we were home by about
ten-thirty p.m. and I went straight to bed. I found I had
difficulty sleeping, and I tossed to get comfortable. I
also felt the bulge around my waist expanding, and
soon none of my clothes fit. Before long, I weighed in at
200 pounds, a thirty-five-pound increase from what I
weighed when I retired in 1999. Among our New Year's
resolutions in 2004, we vowed to eat earlier. My wife
now only takes jobs on Sundays that allow her to get off
no later than eight p.m.

I like to sleep in a warmer room with a minimum
of covers and clothing. I usually wear my Fruit of the
Loom briefs or BVDs (i.e., briefs as opposed to boxers)
and a t-shirt or tank top. In colder weather, I may wear
a baseball shirt (with long-sleeves). I prefer to sleep
with just one sheet and no warm covers. I have trouble
enough maneuvering the one sheet! On some cold
winter nights, however, I have been known to use a

blanket and just struggle a little harder when getting out of bed.

Critical to the whole discipline of sleeping is a clock that is readable at any hour of the night. I have a digital clock with two-inch high numerals, which make the time very clear. When sleeping on vacation or other trips, I try to remember to bring my own time device!

Most all the sleep related activities listed to this point make no reference to any outside help. To this point, by and large, I am able to get into and out of bed on my own. Sometimes my wife (who always goes to bed after me) will take a peek at me to see if I am struggling with any of my many turns. On the bedstead, however, I do keep a call button so that I can alert my wife if I get really locked in. This has efficiently replaced the cowbell that we originally used (and that, incidentally, had the potential to awaken the entire neighborhood!). On occasion, I do sleep on the first floor and I use my cell phone to dial the phone next to her bed when I encountered difficulty.

Also, I have sought the assistance of my good friend Doug Hobby and others, who have helped me negotiate the stairs from our living room to the second-floor bedroom. I am particularly off, it seems, around the nine or ten in the evening, and Doug usually follows me up the stairs, pushing my butt gently to make sure I keep moving up the steps. Momentum is an important part of the process, and Doug makes sure I don't stop along the way! Once I am in bed, Doug sits and watches a little late evening baseball or basketball with me. I am very fortunate to have a friend like Doug.

My neurologist, Dr. Cheryl Waters, was concerned that my sleepless nights might be starting to weaken me, affecting my energy level and overall health. She prescribed amitriptyline, a sleeping pill, and suggested one or two tablets per evening depending how they impacted my sleep. I resisted, but finally I conceded and began to take half a sleeping pill. I had never taken a sleeping pill before, and I was a bit nervous about its impact.

After I took my first pill, I found that it was indeed effective, and I slept comfortably for the balance of the evening. However, upon waking up, I had a floating feeling, as if I were drifting straight to heaven. I imagined that the guys in the white sheets were on their way to take me to the promised land. It was a feeling which I had never experienced before, and I felt like the end was near. For several months, the half pill a day was the only sampling I made from Dr. Waters's prescription.

As my defensive maneuvers to gain more rest at night proved unsuccessful, I again turned to the sleeping pill as a possible source of some sustained sleeping time. My wife divided a pill from her inventory of Tylenol PM, and I found that this procedure helped me sleep for longer periods of time. Eventually, I again worked my way into the pills prescribed by Dr. Waters.

Although I was reluctant to add another category of pills to my already bulky intake, the possibility of correcting my sleep discomfort was worth the chance.

The sleep factor contains yet another frustrating aspect of living with Parkinson's and being retired. Theoretically, I should have lots of time for reading all those books I received for Father's Day and Christmas over the years. Recently, I met up with Peter Simon, who I met through my Lafayette College connection years ago. Peter is the son of the late William E. Simon, former secretary of the treasury and energy czar in the Ford and Nixon administrations. He was a candidate for vice president at the Republican National Convention when President Gerald Ford selected Bob Dole instead.

Like his father, Peter started his business career as a bond trader but specialized more in convertible (corporate) bonds rather than municipals and governments. When I met Peter, I was involved with corporates more than munies, and also we were linked by a common membership in the Delta Tau Delta Fraternity. When we reunited recently, he expressed an interest in my book entitled *Howard Powerless,* and befitting of our backgrounds, we arranged a swap. Peter offered me a copy of his father's autobiography in trade for one of my *Howard* books.

I jumped into the Simon biography as soon as it arrived at my doorstep. However, as I read on, I found myself constantly falling asleep while reading. I had the same experience while reading the biography of Lafayette and John Grisham's *The Last Juror.* Not only did I fall sound asleep, I had some mishaps in the course of my reading. For example, about a hundred pages into the Simon book, I took a sip of coffee and fell asleep before I could put the cup down on the table. Within a short span of time, I was pouring the coffee down the center of my Bermuda shorts and onto the pages of my new book. Fortunately, I am not a fan of piping hot coffee or I would have burned myself pretty badly.

In another incident, while reading the Lafayette biography to pass the time while getting a pedicure, I fell asleep and dropped my book into the tub at my feet. There is no drifting off phase evident any of my book reading experiences. I wonder if it has to do with my forming a mental image from my reading and then transferring this image into a dream-like state. Almost any time I am reading along, I find myself dropping the book onto the floor. I probably will have to buy a book holder!

Unfortunately, although the Parkinson's disease routine is the same every day, the victim cannot just put his or her solution on auto pilot and expect to comfortably adjust to life's continuously changing circumstances. Focus is so important, and often lost in the repetitive nature of our answer to our problems. For example, one morning I awoke thinking it was time for my jump start first serving of the day's pills. Without checking my clock, I quickly sat up and downed the four pills that normally start my day around six a.m. I had awakened feeling pretty good, and was ready to tackle the day. My mood was soon dampened, however, when I turned my head and looked at the clock. It wasn't even five a.m.—the time read 4:54. In effect, I had underslept! And I couldn't unswallow the pills. After dealing with PD for more than twelve years, this was the first time I had mistimed my daily opener. This daily opener is the potion which liberates us—more or less—every day! I knew it would result in several freeze-ups during the day, but I decided to stretch out the time units to 3.5 hours instead. My first freeze-up occurred at eight-thirty a.m. and lasted about thirty minutes. It felt like the pills I took at eight-thirty a.m. (normally slated for nine a.m.) were slow to take effect. With some strain, I was able to type at the word processor from about eight-forty-five a.m. Fortunately, I had nothing planned for the morning—no golf, no doctors meetings, or other important plans, and so the incident was not all that disruptive. "Focus" became my new motto in life.

On the flip side, it doesn't seem to help my demeanor to oversleep the five-forty-five to six o'clock self-imposed deadline. In September 2004, I had an awful night trying to sleep, as perceived financial problems and a host of other matters started to work on my psyche around one a.m. In particular, trying to work out the seating arrangements for the more than 200 guests expected at my daughter's wedding reception in about forty-five days seemed to be filled with unexpected conflicts! At any rate, around five-thirty a.m., I must have finally relaxed and I fell sound asleep. When I awoke, my large clock read 6:45, and I was frozen solid. Even when I tried the maneuvers listed above (i.e. moving any part of my body just to get rolling), I couldn't get my body to respond. My bladder was stirring, so I felt a sense of urgency. I somehow got my body into a makeshift position and I was able to take the pills I should have consumed more than an hour earlier. With an extreme amount of physical effort, I was able to slide my body so that I was seated on the bed. Even so, each thrust I made toward the edge of the bed seemed to gain only a quarter of an inch along the way. Finally, I rang the alarm to signal my wife that I needed help getting started on the day. She wasn't too concerned about me because just two days prior, I had pulled myself from bed, dressed, and descended the stairs without waking her throughout the entire process. But this particular morning, she monitored my every step and ultimately I made it to the bathroom and back, got dressed and cleaned up, and headed for the first floor of our house.

On this particular morning, too, the stairs seemed somewhat intimidating. The tension from my freeze-up caused my hands to perspire and to stick to the banister as I made my way. My knees were still very tight and showed little or no bend. I proceeded very gradually, but didn't stop along the way. My wife followed me down the stairs and helped me get seated in my wheelchair once I was all the way down. She guided me into the kitchen and I soon became relaxed as I had some orange juice and doughnuts. Before taking any food, though, I exhaled a huge amount of breath. My ordeal of the morning was over.

Perhaps the most depressing part of Parkinson's disease is the matter of being unable to drive a car. At least four drivers have volunteered on a regular basis to take me to my various destinations. As illustrated in the above example of dropping my coffee on the Simon book, driving a car is not allowed because I can fall asleep without any advance warning. Before I came to this realization, one time, while driving on curvaceous Parsonage Hill Road, I drifted off and when I realized what was happening, I found myself driving on the *opposite shoulder* before I snapped out of it and could pull my car back to its proper lane. Cars with which I could have had a life-threatening head-on collision had swung off the busy connecting road between Chatham and Short Hills. They were literally on the edge of the swamp that engulfs the road at the point of my near accident.

On other occasions, the grooved shoulders on Route 78 woke me up as I drifted off. I remember my pal Hobby screaming at me to wake up while on the way home from a golf match. Even short drives—to someplace just a few blocks away like the pharmacy or the post office—are not advisable if there are traffic lights to negotiate. I have found myself starting to fall asleep at these lights while waiting for them to change. My latest trick is to put the car in neutral or park, and apply the emergency brake until the green light comes on. But other than occasional short distances, I just don't drive.

I have also mentioned the slowness on the right side of my body. My ability to move my right foot from the accelerator to the brake in a sudden stop is definitely impaired.

Sleeping during the day also has made me less than a solid performer on any committees on which I might serve. If I attend a seminar, I am apt to fall asleep during discussion of any topic that is less than exciting. I like to take notes, but my handwriting is so awful that I can barely make out even a few words. My best times are during mid-morning (say, nine-thirty until noon). Very early and after lunch are definitely a struggle for me.

I recently participated in a full day of activities relating to Volunteer Day for Lafayette College. This is a day when alumni are recognized for their actions on behalf of the college. A scrumptious lunch, extensive awards to the outstanding alumni of the college for their volunteer efforts, and speeches from some top college officials were all part of the program from noon until about two p.m. The off-site location, the Nassau Inn in Princeton, was alluring and added to the adventure of the day. After lunch, we headed for our respective break-out sessions (i.e., dedicated to special purposes), and specialized training on fund raising and use of the class Web site. As the Web administrator for the Class of 1960, I should have been especially dialed in on the content for this session. My fellow Class of 1960 alums grabbed front row seats and so I pulled my walker alongside their area. About ten minutes into the session, however, I found myself drifting off, and I was conspicuous to the speaker because I kept dropping my pen and notebook onto the floor. Try as I might, I just couldn't keep my eyes open! I fought the tape and finally seemed to snap out of my trance after about twenty minutes of nodding. I closed strong, and even asked questions before the session ended at four p.m. I hoped that Debbie Cummings, the session leader, understood my dilemma.

Another difficulty that has arisen out of this form of narcolepsy affects my ability to efficiently self publish my writings. Constant proofreading is required in the field of publishing, and I just cannot stay with my manuscripts long enough to ensure a flawless product. Hopefully, my writings will not put you or any outside editors to sleep as well!

With the advance in my Parkinson's condition, and the change in my sleeping habits, I have noticed fewer vivid dreams. My concerns about potential financial difficulties seem to swirl through my mind when I am trying to sleep at night. During the day, when I can look at my overall financial plan, I tend to stop worrying or make some adjustment in the plan. To "pinch myself" in the middle of the night, I often turn on the TV set for about fifteen minutes and that makes the financial nightmares disappear.

When traveling, an unfamiliar bed at a hotel or motel adds to the complications of a PD patient. In the case of a twin-bedded room, I am apt to select the bed closest to the bathroom. Also, because I sleep with a minimum of covers, I try to pick the bed furthest from any window. I set up an end table with my pills and a bottle of water close at hand. I usually set up my walker somewhere between my sleeping location and the bathroom. When I remove my shoes, I try to place them within reach to facilitate my initial move the next day. I try to retire with the bathroom light on but the door partially open. This gives me a target when I have to get up in the middle of the night.

On a related subject, I used to like lying out in the sun—sometimes falling asleep—and obtaining a bit of a suntan. But in recent years, because I tense up so dramatically when I sleep, I find that when I awake from sleeping in the sun I feel just terrible and can hardly move. Those at the pool or at the beach see me struggling to catch my bearings, and my actions can startle them. Now I usually pick out partially shaded areas and sit and read or write at a table with a straight-back chair. In the tropics of Florida and the Caribbean, you can soak up a lot of incidental sun without sitting out in the open. Besides, too much exposure to the sun isn't good for you anyway!

Occasionally, while traveling on an overnight trip with the likes of Doug Hobby or Raymond Monroe, I have the chance to call on someone other than my wife to help me find the bathroom in the middle of the night. Usually, I find the guys I travel with to be supportive of my efforts to get out of bed at two a.m., although they're not altogether happy with the idea. In general, they help me out and quickly return to bed and back to sleep. In my wife's case, she usually likes to give me a little incentive to not wake her up again. She likes to say, "I guess I will see you in a couple of hours," implying that I will again be calling on her to help at four a.m.

Also, I find that the guys tend to put the middle of the night trip behind them, while my wife likes to tell her girlfriends about how bad my evening was. Other than writing this memo, I rarely think about my restless nights.

After successfully completing the election of officers at the 2004 annual meeting, eight members of the board of governors of the Bond Club of NJ decided to play the Morris County Country Club layout. I had a modest interest in playing, but that would have created an odd number of players. So I elected to ride along in a single cart and to join up with whichever foursome was moving faster. I tried hitting the ball a few times, and suddenly I was overcome by a huge freeze-up. I was able to maneuver the cart, although not with confidence, as the course was extremely hilly. Around the ninth hole, I had to go to the bathroom and Bryan Walter—my former business partner—had to escort me to the men's room located in the back of the halfway house. The other golfers had never seen me need such assistance before, and the expressions on their collective faces reflected a deep concern for my condition.

Upon completion of my duties in the men's room, there was a chorus of offers to take me back to the club house, but I assured them all that my PD medicine would soon take hold and that I would be fine for the remainder of the day. Five holes later, I took the driver from the bag and faced the prospect of trying to hit a 185–yard par three. My first shot went left about twenty yards. One of the governors, John Blum I believe, said, "Hit another one." And the second or Mulligan drive landed just two feet short of the green. I chipped on, two putted, and recorded an adjusted bogey on the hole. I also bogeyed the seventeenth hole without the benefit of a Mulligan, as I almost drove the green with my time-tested one iron.

On the eighteenth hole, my second shot was a beautiful five-iron shot, straight down alongside the pond, which placed me well ahead of the others who were busy searching the woods and the water for their drives. Having to wait to hit my next shot, I fell fast asleep in the middle of the eighteenth fairway. Suddenly, I heard several of the governors yelling at me, "Paul, are you all right?" I am sure they thought I was dead! Once awake, I hit my third shot poorly and then chipped on the green to finish my day of golf. I think I was enough of a distraction for this group.

After a few weeks of physical training with the MARA group, I began to notice that I was sleeping more soundly. I surmised that the exercise was helpful in tiring me out just enough to force me to sleep. The exercise whereby I stood up from a sitting position on a beach ball helped me spring from (1) the bed and (2) the toilet seat. The training seemed to coincide with a reduced incidence of my calling on help in the middle of the night. My wife was very pleased with this development.

Part of my more pleasant bedtime activities involved my confidence in getting up in the middle of the night just to stretch out after sleeping so long (and ultimately freezing up) in a fixed position. Arising in the middle of the night also enabled me to enjoy the Sinemet CR high that kicked in about three a.m.! Far be it for me to explain why this pill taken at bedtime would influence my behavior pattern for five hours (say from ten p.m. to three a.m.) after consumption, but have an impact in sixty to ninety minutes when taken at four-fifteen a.m.!

For most healthy human beings, sleep is accomplished without any special focus or organizational structure. But for me, it is impossible to just get into bed naturally. My actions must be premeditated. Like other matters affecting a Parkinson's victim, sleeping well must be addressed and worked out to each individual's best advantage.

I think I will go take a nap.

Fraternizing with the younger traders enabled me to capture the "esprit" of Wall Street. I realize now that I should have focused more on matters pertaining to my health and well being, but I can't turn back the clock.

Chapter 4

Remaining Socially Active

As a New York Jets syndicate season ticket holder for almost ten years, I have recently benefited from the organization's policies and practices with respect to handicapped spectators. Premiere parking facilities at Giants Stadium (ironically named, even though the Jets play all their home games there) are available to those with cars exhibiting the blue-and-white handicapped stickers issued by New Jersey. Parking attendants seem to jump at the opportunity to help fans with stickers, giving them easy access to the parking spots nearest to the stadium entrance. In many cases, an attendant will wave the car exhibiting said sticker through, allowing it to pass a line of ten or more cars. A special gate for handicapped fans and their helpers leads directly to the wide section behind lower level section 117. Inside the stadium, ample wheelchair space and a folding chair are provided for each handicapped person. These seats are also close to restroom facilities. The handicapped seats are under the cover of the second tier balcony, so I never worry if any precipitation is in the works. The

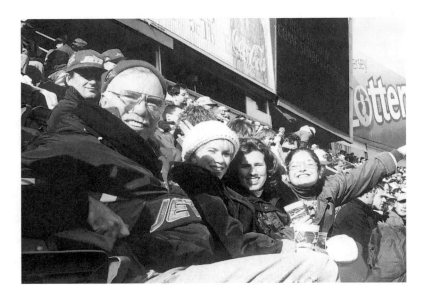

only hassle that can come from the 76,000-plus fans is that you can get bumped around a bit at the crunch time immediately before the game and shortly after the final whistle. Arriving early and leaving after the crowd has dispersed are all part of my strategy.

Major college teams also maintain or should maintain such facilities. Inside its Rutgers Athletic Center (a.k.a. the RAC), Rutgers University has a special elevated section immediately behind the south corner of the arena. To me, they're some of the best seats in the house. Last season, we saw a thriller when Rutgers upset the Syracuse Orangemen in a Big East match-up. Parking at the RAC is relatively close to the gym. Princeton University, on the other hand, puts its handicapped areas quite some distance from the entrance, and the PD

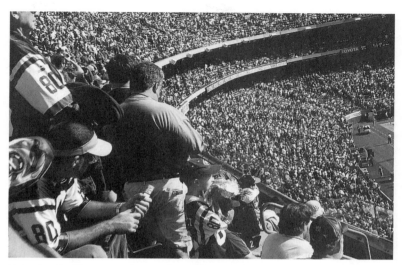

Jets football games draw about 76,999 fans. Author Luscombe sat approximately nine rows from the top of Giants Stadium as shown with his daughter Alison, Erica Cutler Fitzgerald, and Kate Russel Majestro. Being "just nine rows from God" led to Luscombe applying for seats down lower and nearer to the entranceway. (Photo Credit: anonymous JET fan)

victim must negotiate all sorts of sidewalk gradations before reaching the relatively new Jadwin arena.

Princeton's comparatively new football stadium is an architectural beauty, featuring a Roman style that incorporates the original columns from Palmer Stadium. The handicapped parking area for football games is about the same as for basketball games—it requires a long walk and the PD victim must walk the full distance of the field because only one end of the stadium is open to take tickets. When I attended a game there in September 2004, none of the security agents could explain to me why only one end of the stadium was open.

Also, once inside the stadium, the same lack of knowledge on the part of the security personnel prevailed. Not only did I have to walk an extra 150 yards, but also I had to carry my walker up a flight of stairs to get to where I could watch the game. My back and legs hurt for days following the unfriendly experience at Princeton Stadium.

Probably in recognition of my long dedication to its athletic program, Lafayette College has gone out of its way to make me comfortable at football and basketball games. Recently at home basketball games, the sports information director encouraged me to sit at the scorers table whenever there was a vacancy. The specter of a player diving for a loose ball about to go out-of-bounds at my seat crossed my mind, but I fearlessly watched at least ten games from that vantage point. Literally, one of the first seats available as you enter the east side of the basketball arena, I am able to easily negotiate my walker (equipped with a seat) into position. As an aside, because I was in complete view of almost everyone at the game, the special scorers seat helped me reconnect with some old classmates and resurrect my Alumni Column, which I write for the Class of 1960.

In any case, there is no reason for the hardened sports fans to miss any public events because of Parkinson's disease. My main problems arise with little things, like in which pocket did I put my game ticket! Also, the bathroom facilities are a bit untidy by the start of the second quarter.

Actually, some sporting events requiring extensive walking may be difficult to handle. When I play golf now, I must ride in a cart. In fact, my cart has yellow or blue colored flags that not only advertise my handicapped condition but also allow me to park very close to the green.

Though this is often not possible when the course has been saturated by recent rain storms. Sometimes I find I can get a special Parkinson's ruling from one of my playing partners. It is not unusual for any golfer to hit the ball in an area not reachable by cart. Sand traps are one example of an area not reachable by cart.

If the trap is very awkward to negotiate by foot, many of my playing partners let me hit from a level section of the trap without penalty. Or they may allow me to hit from the left side of the fairway if the water on the right side precludes negotiation by cart. Although it is not golf at its purest, my friends seem willing to bend the rules a little bit just to get me out on the course. In my opinion, golf is like a form of therapy that enables me to live a better lifestyle.

Actually attending professional golf tournaments is next to impossible in a cart. Over the years, for example, I have attended at least ten U.S. Open Golf tournaments, including such fine tracks as Baltusrol, Winged Foot, Merion, Shinnecock, Ridgewood, and Saukun Valley. I also marshaled at the NFL Golf Classic, a regular stop on the Seniors Tour and usually held at the somewhat convenient Upper Montclair Country Club.

Although several courses locally have sponsored such events, I have gracefully declined all invitations since my PD reached its advanced stage.

The evolution of stadium golf undoubtedly offers provisions for the handicapped fan, but I have yet to participate in one of these events.

Remaining socially active as a Parkinsonian entails some sacrifices, but the rewards of camaraderie far outweigh the temporary hurt of such activities.

Recently, my wife Cinnie and I celebrated our fortieth wedding anniversary—on April 17, 2004. Cinnie and I met in the early 1960s when each of us had our own apartment in New York City. My lifelong friend Doug Hobby and I were roommates and we had a small apartment on 69th Street near Columbus Avenue, which is now part of the Lincoln Center Complex.

Cinnie had a rotation of about four roommates and lived at 952 Fifth Avenue near 76th Street. When Doug and I decided to hold a St. Patrick's Day party on March 17, 1963, we invited all the females we knew, especially groups of women. We were interested in critical mass! We telephoned Linda Silvestri, whose friends and acquaintances at a Columbia University dorm might inflate the numbers. And we invited Cinnie, hoping for some extra roommate tagalongs. Cinnie came to the party alone, and after a few introductions, I asked her if she would like a drink.

"Do you have any Scotch?" she asked.

Doug Hobby looked at me uneasily, and then I recalled we had about half a pint of Clan McGregor scotch (i.e., one of the cheaper brands then on the market) stashed away in one of our kitchen cabinets. That was probably the extent of our non-beer liquor supply!

"Yes we do," I responded. "Would you like it on the rocks with some club soda?"

"Thank you, that would be fine," she responded

While Doug fetched some ice cubes from the ice tray in the freezer, I had the brilliant idea of adding one of the green color dye tablets to Cinnie's scotch so as to be consistent with all of those drinking St. Pattie's Day green beer. Doug supported the idea. We didn't want her to feel out of place at such a major social event!

Although the green scotch may have been repulsive to the classic scotch drinker, Cinnie was a good sport and played along with the gag.

And so our relationship began with a green scotch! The rest of the story is written in history. Shortly after the green scotch party, Cinnie and I started dating and usually our dinners out involved some sort of alcohol. Thirteen months later we were married. Cinnie never abandoned her taste for scotch, upgrading from the likes of Clan McGregor to Dewars. I liked scotch (Grants then Dewars) for a while, and changed over to martinis sometime in the 1980s. After some warnings from the family doctor, I converted entirely to white wine around 1990. With the onset of Parkinson's, I decided to give up drinking entirely.

In part, my policy about alcohol stems from the warnings listed on the labels of certain of my regular Parkinson's medicine. For example, both mirapex and comtan carry warnings about the PD patient's use of alcohol. Their specific words are: "Alcohol may intensify effect." Now, during any cocktail hour, my drink is O'-Doul's nonalcoholic beer, the exception being that, on occasion, I do sip some white crème de menthe at meetings of the Chatham Mens Club. For dessert, I seem addicted to vanilla ice cream with a shot of green crème de menthe poured over. As time has passed, I have started to have a glass or two of chardonnay at dinnertime. I frequently leave the first glass unfinished.

The evenings spent with the Mens Club have been a very important part of my daily living experience.

Originally, the Club consisted of Ken Thompson and Doug Hobby, who dropped by the house to watch a significant sporting event. On one occasion—on March 9, 2001—Ken and Doug came over to watch the college basketball playoff game between Holy Cross and Navy, and they consumed a few cocktails, ate shrimp hors d'oeuvres, and ultimately ordered a pizza from nearby Romanelli's. We were treated to an exciting overtime win by Holy Cross! But around eight p.m. I noticed my legs starting to stiffen and so I passed along the responsibility of attending to the pizza man when the doorbell rang. I had anticipated my rigidity and had the fifteen dollars cash on hand for Ken to pay the delivery man. My pockets are constantly filled with five- and ten-dollar bills as an alternative to trying to finger the right currency from my wallet when such situations arise.

Doug and I easily consumed three slices of the cheese pizza, while Ken (the skinny guy among us) had the remaining two slices. Our luxurious meal was rounded out with raspberry flavored Popsicles. Indeed, the scene reminded us of the commercial slogan, "It doesn't get any better than this."

Upon her return from her job at the PaperMill Playhouse, my wife immediately criticized us for the lack of balance in our meal. I accused her of trying to run an inquisition about our evening, but in the future I assured her that we would order salads with our pizza.

As time passed by, the Chatham Mens Club expanded its horizons beyond watching sporting events on TV. We developed a keen interest in competitive card games, most important of which were Skip-Bo and Sequences. The games were intense and mentally stimulating.

When my wife and I were feted at our fortieth wedding anniversary party, I expected to have maybe two or three O'Doul's throughout the course of the evening. The affair was held in nearby downtown Chatham at Danniello's Restaurant, which has no liquor license. Nonetheless, Daneallo's provides elegant wine buckets for the patron to use when his or her own alcoholic beverage has been brought. My preference for nonalcoholic beer and O'Doul's was accommodated and my wife imported her scotch in an Evian bottle. Others brought red or white wine, depending on their personal taste or expected entrée. Once the cocktail set-up had been accomplished, there was little room on the table for anything else! My seat was right in front of one of the refill buckets for white wine where, during the course of the evening, my daughters Alison and Priscilla were constantly refilling the white wine glasses of the dozen or so guests. Soon I could no longer resist temptation, and so I tried a glass of the white wine nestled in the ice right in front of me. As I raised the bottle, I noticed the brand was Turning Leaf Reserve, a California chardonnay. Upon sampling the wine, I found it quite savory and before long I was on my second glass. Over the past few years, most white wines have tasted bitter to me and—before this anniversary party—I couldn't remember when I had finished a glass. Then came glasses three and four, then possibly even a fifth. Suddenly, I felt I was reenacting the country music hit about José Cuervo!

An invisible force seemed to sustain my body movements and my normal trend toward rigidity at nine in the evening seemed to subside. Suddenly I was on my feet chatting with the guests at the opposite end of the table. I stood and talked with them for a longer time than I would have anticipated. Then I took a little walk outside with my daughter Alison. It was a beautiful night and we felt we needed some fresh air. A little after ten p.m., I suggested it was time for me to go before I started to wear my true PD colors. I signaled to Raymond Monroe, our designated driver, to prepare to leave and quickly he had his bright red Ford Explorer parked in front of the restaurant, literally thirty yards from my seat at the party. Within minutes, my wife and I were on board and headed for our house some ten blocks away.

As mentioned herein, on most evenings I stiffen up somewhat dramatically after ten o'clock. But still I felt like some sort of strange power—the unmoved mover perhaps—was helping me the night of our fortieth. Upon arriving home, I headed for the stairs and, unassisted, proceeded to get ready for bed.

Unlike most nights, I quickly undressed, went to the bathroom, brushed my teeth, and hopped into bed. The feeling was awesome. I fell asleep fairly quickly.

When I awoke some two hours later, around twelve-thirty, I realized I was no longer cured of Parkinson's disease. My short-lived pleasant experience had disappeared and rigidity had returned. Quite stiff, I wanted to test my ability to get to the adjacent bathroom. I could hear someone in the bathroom down the hall. I assumed it was our daughter Priscilla—a resident of Alexandria, Virginia—who was staying overnight with us. I beckoned her to my side with a subtle whistle, and soon she was in my bedroom to help. We lined up a route using various props and she helped me get to and from the bathroom. We discussed the dehydrating impact of the wine, and so I drank a fair amount of water before returning to bed. Once back in bed, I had difficulty in rotating back to the position whereby I was facing the exit from the bed. I felt as if the wine was weakening my mental resolve and/or my physical power to extricate myself from the bed. Also, I realized I had done no planning about my next day's attire. I was literally miles from any change of clothes!

After these initial concerns, I did end up sleeping fairly soundly. I awoke and awkwardly took my CR pill about four-twenty-five. I calculated the impact of the pill would hit about six a.m., exactly when I would be taking my opening salvo of medicine for the day. But I slept right through the CR and woke up at a little after six. I took my jump starter portion (which included four pills), but I didn't feel the impact for another forty-five minutes. Also, I needed some help from my wife to get dressed and to get moving in the direction of our living room. She lined up some shorts for me to wear and helped me lift myself up from the bed. I continue to be amazed at how strong she is!

Once I had breakfast, the day after the anniversary party was essentially uneventful. I sat at the computer and wrote a few pages of a manuscript for more than two hours. Perhaps, I thought, I would dabble in a little wine at dinner that night—maybe one or two glasses—to see if it would make my life a little more tolerable.

My Nutley (New Jersey) high school graduation class has been very active, with three or four reunions per year. That's right, *per year!* Possibly the first class to graduate to the recording of *Graduation Day* by the then popular vocal group The Four Lads, the Nutley High School Class of 1956 has an organizational structure that regularly schedules gatherings at restaurants within the Nutley environs. Many are at restaurants that we used to patronize when we were teenagers (e.g., Rutts Hutt and Mario's). As the Class prepares more actively for its fiftieth reunion in 2006, it seems that more and more classmates are getting interested in the location and slate of activities for the affair. The group is spearheaded by Ron Kulik, who every August sponsors a summer barbeque at his home on Long Beach Island. Former Penn State University football placement kicker Sam Stellatella catches a ton of photographs and always seems to have one waiting for you in the mail a few days after the function.

Interest in the reunions seemed to intensify in the aftermath of September 11, 2001. It seems almost anyone in New Jersey had a contemporary, relative, or neighbor who perished in the World Trade Center tragedy. When I retired from Morgan Stanley in 1999, I had an office on the sixtieth floor of WTC #2. Fortunately, none of my immediate coworkers (to my knowledge) died in the collapse of the tower. However, in Chatham, two of my neighbors (Dennis Buckley and Don Adams) perished along with scores of employees of the Cantor Fitzgerald Corporation. It seemed that our mini-reunions provided a form of therapy for those directly or closely impacted by the events of 9/11.

Over the past few years, despite my PD, I have been able to participate in these functions with more or less distinction. Most recently, my wife drove me to the event at the Red Robin Restaurant on Route 3 East in Clifton. Totally out of character, we arrived twenty minutes before the seven p.m. advertised start time for the party. We were fortunate to line up a favorable location for the evening and we could also socialize with the class officers who were there early to ensure that everything was well organized. This was a much more favorable experience than when we are late and have to squeeze in to the last remaining seats. Or be stuck miles from the men's room! Also, by arriving early, we could gracefully leave early!

However, my experiences at some of the other Class of 1956 mini-reunions have not been quite so smooth.

At the summer meeting in 2003, I was stranded in a crowded section of the party when I felt the need to head home. Somehow you instinctively feel your total system is about to shut down and you know your body will probably go into an extended off position. I confided in one of my favorite classmates—"Bunny" Wilcox Jenkins—and she collected two or three of the more physical members at the party and they helped me wind my way through the crowd, literally with one of them under each of my shoulders. Once I got to my car, and my wife was ready, we were on our way to our next destination.

In March of 2002, John "Hank" Olson and his wife Sandy drove me to the class function. As a precaution, we loaded my wheelchair into their SUV. The party was to be at Mario's Restaurant, which is where many of us bought our first slice of pizza ever! The turnout was yet another success and the evening flew by. The event was the first one following the tragic events of September 11, 2001. Hank was fortunate to escape from his office at Morgan Stanley on the sixty-sixth floor of WTC #2. Eleanor Schmidt, another classmate, was there—she lost many coworkers from the Fiduciary Trust Company. She was lucky to be alive—she simply was late for work that morning. Unfortunately, captivated by all the stories circulating that evening, I didn't pay attention to time or my pill period, and before I knew it, I was sinking into a significant Parkinson's funk. It was too late to counter the trend, and as Ron Kulik made his closing remarks, I knew I would be on display as the Class Zombie. I glanced around the room that Mario's had set aside for us, and I couldn't find Hank. My anxiety eased as soon Hank returned from the quieter area of the restaurant where he had been phoning his daughter in the Poconos. When Hank asked me what the problem was, I informed him I was experiencing a freeze-up and probably would have to use my wheelchair to get to his SUV. Hank nodded and quickly went to his vehicle to fetch the wheelchair. Again, my exit was fairly conspicuous.

My best friend Doug Hobby frequently says, "Luscombe, we can't take you anywhere!" Although he is probably right, Doug still encourages me to circulate, and he frequently forces the issue by making golf starting times without my knowledge. When he says he has a time on a given date, I usually agree to join him.

On a smaller scale, I try to have lunch out at a restaurant as often as possible. Bob Faig, a stockbroker with Wachovia Securities (he's originally from the Prudential Bache side), is my most regular lunch companion. Bob is approximately ten years older than I, but has no apparent health problems. He still exhibits a smooth, powerful golf swing and enjoys the BCNJ golf outings. Professionally, he teams up with his son Chuck at the local Short Hills office for Wachovia, and the twosome has been very effective in finding high yield instruments for my IRA. We enjoy our lunches and he usually brings research material on one or two of my holdings, or we just talk about the overall performance of my portfolio. Sometimes we even discuss macroeconomics, but Bob prefers talking about the market and individual companies. He has his one gin martini, with an olive, straight up almost every time we dine. I envy his selection—I used to drink Absolute vodka martinis before 1990.

These lunches with Bob Faig and others are therapeutic. They allow me to participate in the "real world" and get me out of the house. For any luncheon, golf outing, conference, or dinner, it entails getting dressed up, showering and shaving, and combing my hair! Without a social excuse, it is so easy to let oneself go and ignore one's appearance.

I must confess that a degree of anxiety overcomes me before attending any social event, particularly if the venue is somewhere unfamiliar or if the gathering is apt to extend into the night. I constantly try to talk myself out of attending when my off cycle roughs me up during the day. I get very negative, and envision falling like I did at the golf outing where I won the $830 raffle. Often my friend Raymond plays a role in situations like this. He lectures me on the advantages of going out, tells me that I am a real "go-getter," and to hurry up and get ready! His positive attitude is important to me and my life.

During the winter months, my pal Doug Hobby includes me in his monthly golf luncheon group, at least before most of the group disperses to their winter retreats in Florida and other points south. Bob Palmer, Bill May, and Vinnie are all either part of Doug's original engineering professional society or friends of Palmer. Bill May is involved with a barbershop quartet that performs in concerts and contests. Naturally, the luncheon group supports the concerts. Doug's group consistently takes me to new restaurants and different parts of northern New Jersey.

Fraternizing with the younger traders on Wall Street has enabled me to think and feel younger. As a bond salesman, I always considered the traders to be my most valuable allies and, at the peak of my business career, I spent many a Thursday night on the social circuit with them.

With most of my contemporaries more interested in their retirement plans and medical insurance, or even worse their specific ailments, I was more interested in the 'esprit' of the youth that tended to surround me at Prudential Bache, Alex Brown, and Dean Witter (subsequently Morgan Stanley). I realize now that I should have focused more on matters pertaining to my health and well-being, but I can't turn back the clock.

I still encourage contact with the younger sector of our society. One of my best friends is Ken Thompson, a thirty-two-year-old neighbor of mine whose father died when he was just ten years old. Together we have seen every type of sporting event imaginable, including David Cone's perfect game against the Montreal Expos in the summer of 2000. We were one of a handful of fans who braved the February cold to witness two XFL football games at the Meadowlands. Outdoors! (Note: The XFL failed at the end of that season.) We have exchanged birthday and Christmas presents for years. Usually I receive something related to the NY Jets and he gets something emblematic of his beloved Dolphins.

Ken also enjoys the restaurant chain known as Hooters. We have tried several of these restaurants along the eastern seaboard. They feature somewhat scantily clad young waitresses who are very friendly. Their typical uniform is a snug white tank top tucked into a pair of short cropped orange shorts. (See the picture from the Rockville, Maryland Hooters.) Recently, as I was recovering from my emergency appendectomy, Ken encouraged me to try out the new Hooters restaurant on Route 22 in Union. At the age of sixty-five and sporting a cane,

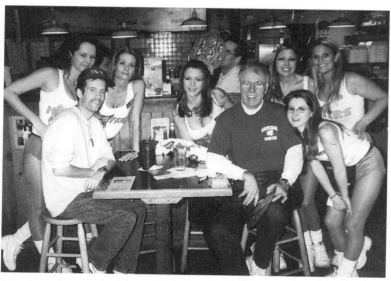

Ken Thompson and author Paul Luscombe enjoy the "Hooters" Restaurant in Rockville, MD. The two sports fans were en route to see Lafayette College play in the Patriot League basketball tourney in nearby Upper Marlboro.

I had to be the oldest person in the restaurant. Our waitress felt right at home and sat at our table while she took down our order. Her tank top had to be at least one size too small! We had a blast! I totally forgot about my Parkinson's disease and had a great time!

In the mid 1990s, I had occasion to visit with Ken at the Vernon Ski Lodge in northern New Jersey. We had a full night of cocktailing planned, and following a dinner at the Four Season's Restaurant, we hit one of the bars servicing the lobby personnel. It was then that Ken introduced me to the art of doing shots, which was a means of attaining an instant state of intoxication. Shots were symbolic of the in-a-hurry mentality of the late 1980s and early 1990s. My contemporaries are more inclined to drink beer and on some occasions a 7 and 7 (i.e., Seagrams 7 brand rye with 7–Up soda). As we did our five or six shots of Yeagomeister liquor, it was almost as if I could feel the alcohol go directly to my brain. The next day, I felt awful. When I looked at the credit card receipt, I was not only disturbed by the size of the bill, but also by the illegible scribble representing my signature. It resembled a "flat-liner" cardio chart! Perhaps some brain damage that exaggerated my PD resulted from the evening in New Vernon.

Keeping a full social schedule necessitates keeping one's appearance up to high standards. For example, shaving and showering are a must and I get a haircut once a month. I prefer a shorter haircut because it's low maintenance. I usually go to the franchise known as Hair Core, where the rate for a shampoo and haircut is fourteen dollars. When I initially sit in the barber's chair, my guy usually asks me how I would like my hair done. I quickly tell him, "Buzz size 5," which is the middle level for the various buzz attachments that he has. The procedure takes about five minutes and I am soon almost ready to join the Marines!

In general, I have to be careful of spilling food and drinks, or simply knocking over glassware at any of my social events. When I order my O'Doul's non-alcoholic beer, I send back the frosted tall glass and drink straight from the bottle. Tall beer glasses are just too tipsy! At buffet dinners, I usually allow my wife or a friend to fill my plate. My worst incident occurred at Ron Kulik's summer house, at his annual summer party for the Nutley High School Class of 1956. Seated in his recently painted off-white living room, one of my classmates benevolently prepared me a shrimp cocktail laden with the traditional red cocktail sauce. At the time, I was on and should have easily handled the tasty appetizer. However, as my confidence gained some momentum, I soon was in the middle of telling some story and was undoubtedly using my arms to demonstrate a point. Once I had the shrimp cocktail in my hands, I couldn't hold still. As if hurling a discus, I unintentionally sent the shrimp plate on an airborne mission toward Ron's beautiful white walls. They were quickly decorated with red cocktail sauce—it looked like Ron was attempting some sort of modern-art deco.

Fortunately, those nearby formed an ad hoc clean-up committee, springing into action and rinsing down the wall. No long-term damage was done. Now, when offered, I take one shrimp at a time.

One of the most frustrating aspects of PD is the matter of getting dressed when one is not firmly set in the on position. If you are trying to do all the social activities I am suggesting, you probably will have to get dressed for a social occasion when you are in the off position. In the spring of 2004, so as to better organize myself for my expected multiple social activities, I wanted to set aside the pairs of Bermuda shorts and other warm weather apparel which fit me! My new and not-so-improved physique made it essential to try on Bermuda shorts, swim trunks, summer-weight slacks, khakis, and tons of shirts and vests. It was silly to clutter up my room with so many clothes that just didn't fit me. And so the wardrobe testing began.

When I started this project at nine in the morning, I was fairly on and so I started trying on items from this accumulation of clothes. With items that fit around the waist, it was essential to check out the item of clothing in the crotch when I sat down. Quite a few items could slide up over my hips, but failed the sit-down test. The articles that had elasticized waist bands had the best shot.

It was so disappointing to realize how many items didn't fit. Maybe one item in every ten barely made the grade. As the length of time dragged on for this project, my nine a.m. medicines were starting to wear off. Soon, I came to a pair of Bermudas that I had worn just the day before. I knew they would fit! As I tried to pull this pair up over my hips, my arms suddenly froze and I stalled without quite getting my shorts up and over my underwear. Getting angry at myself, I groaned and made a fair amount of noise. Frustrated again! It seems that articles of clothing which are so easy to put on when you are in the on position become difficult in the off position.

My wife could hear the commotion and volunteered, "Can I help?"

"Yes!!!" I blurted out without any of my customary tact.

"I'll be right there," she said. "I just have to wash the dirt off my hands."

"Hurry!!!" I exclaimed, as the pressure on my stiffened knee started to intensify and was very painful. My patience, normally regarded as one of my virtues, was growing thin.

"Why does she take so long to wash her hands?" I mumbled under my breath. "She always does a few items for herself ahead of my requirements."

Then a little louder, I said, "My needs come first. I'm the one who's handicapped!"

Undeterred, feeling the need to let out some of the hot air, she proceeded to open the window in the small dressing room and then faced me, ready to help. Although I could tell she was not too pleased with my antics, she worked the difficult shorts up to waist level. She then reminded me of the many items she was working on for me that day, most particularly lunch and dinner.

Once my shorts were in position, I regretted having been so abrupt with my wife. Though rare, I occasionally exhibit a Dr. Jeykel and Mr. Hyde personality. We rarely have two-way verbal disagreements. I just know that the Parkinson's factor exaggerated my estimation of the situation and resulted in my voice being loud and belligerent. I hope she will forgive me.

Being socially active potentially involves having dinner with an out-of-town friend at a fancy New York restaurant. On such occasions, my favorite restaurant is Renee Peugot, a distinctly classical French restaurant located on 51st Street at 8th Avenue. Most of the clients of the restaurant are headed for a Broadway show, but we had indicated to the maître d' that we were in no hurry and would prefer not to rush through dinner.

Once seated, one of the multitude of busboys or assistant waiters was very attentive to our table. He immediately set my friend Charlie and me up with water, bread, and butter, and then he took the time to place the white dinner napkins on each of our laps. Unknown to the waiter, I have a hang-up with dinner napkins stemming from my Parkinson's disease. I simply cannot keep them on my lap! So in the course of dinner, about every three or four minutes, my napkin accidentally slipped to the floor. And there was our waiter, quick on the draw, unfolding a fresh dinner napkin from the stack of clean laundry and proceeding to place it on my lap. I insisted I didn't need a new napkin following each drop, but our waiter had his instructions.

This napkin syndrome was definitely a social skill that I had to work on. To repeat my friend Hobby's assessment, "Luscombe, we can dress you up but we just can't take you anywhere!"

When I saw the American Airlines jet crash into WTC #2, I could almost feel the impact some twenty-three miles away. The plane seemed to accomplish a direct hit on my former desk.

Chapter 5A

Attempts to Continue a Career

To many Parkinson's victims, one of the more difficult aspects in life is accepting the inability to continue working. This forfeiture may not take place immediately, and may be postponed depending on the extent of physical activity required. Some Parkinsonians continue their careers for a long period of time. In my case, I continued to work on Wall Street for seven years from the time I discovered I was stricken. I might have stayed on for a few more years, but instinct told me to call it quits while I was ahead!

From the time I discovered that I had Parkinson's in 1992 until I decided to retire, I maintained an active business schedule in my position at Dean Witter and subsequently Morgan Stanley. I wore the title of Senior Vice President, and my primary function was to cover several mid-sized and medium large sized financial institutions, including some commercial banks, mutual savings banks, investment advisors, large bank trust departments, insurance companies, and a very active hedge fund. Teamed with my partner Bryan Walter, I provided back-up on a second list of accounts. Our clients were competitive, required special service, and tended to move quickly to capitalize on any small differentials in the marketplace. Many accounts were performance oriented, and their relative success versus some predetermined index (such as the ten-year United States Treasury index or the corporate intermediate term bond index) influenced their personal paychecks and the amount of money they retained under management. Most blocks of bonds moved in relatively large increments ($1 million pieces and some many times larger) and all the business was consummated on the telephone. Because the size of these orders was substantial, the slightest errors in price would be compounded into huge numbers of dollars.

Initially, I kept my Parkinson's discovery a secret. I did, however, inform Bryan, with whom I shared commissions. Since ours was not a fifty-fifty split, I felt our ratio should be adjusted to reflect the effectiveness of my sales performance. As far as I could tell, with the possible exception of[1] a sympathy trade, the PD factor

---

[1]Some of the specific names and accounts that I covered were: Chase Bank (Vin Morris, John Rochford, John Schmucker);First Fidelity Bank (Dick Nicholson, Steve Blocklin, George Weckel); Union Carbide Pension (Jim McCabe);Weiss Peck & Grier Advisors (A. Roy Knudsen); Bear Stearns Asset Management (Peter Mahoney, Scott Pavlak); Provident Savings Bank (Kevin Ward, Linda Niro, Ed Reilly); Howard Savings Bank (John Quinn, LeAnne Plunckett); NJ Manufacturers Insurance Co (Peter Bogart); MBL in liquidation (John Quinn); Granite Savings Bank (Charlie Smith, Bill Henson); Peapack Gladstone Bank (Rich Donnelly); Kingswood Growth Fund (Chris Maurizi, Dan Duffy); and Wake Forest University Endowment Fund (John Willard).

did not exactly prompt an increase in business! But I stayed on the payroll and paid very close attention to the details of my job. What was noticeably lost was my ability to whip and drive—get on a roll and knock off several orders at once. In the bond profession, business begets business, and one trade frequently leads to several others. As my Parkinson's factor intensified, I felt myself wrapped up in the minutiae of a trade instead of using it as a wedge to generate more business.

In this mental game of Wall Street numbers trades versus the brain drain that accompanies PD, what seemed odd to me was that I still had the capacity to conceptualize trades and envision methods of improving performance. One of my clients even nicknamed me "Doctor of Bondology" in recognition of my broad understanding of the market. As I grew frustrated by my limitations, I started to write up my ideas and fax them to clients (later I would e-mail my ideas). Some simply summarized the forces at work in the marketplace; others discussed buys and sells of specific securities. Yield curve analysis was also a critical part of the studies. I found myself becoming more of a writer than a telephone salesman. Thus the honing of my writing skills, which had been somewhat dormant since my undergraduate days when I wrote for the Lafayette student newspaper, evolved during this transition period with Parkinson's.

My rigidity was not disruptive enough, early in the game, to limit my personal contact with clients. I encouraged golf dates and luncheon (or dinner) dates with the customers. During the span of my business career, I believed that the best way to be productive and enjoy one's job was to develop relationship business.

My clients were my friends, and remain so following my retirement.

In hindsight, I am glad that I took retirement when I did. My perception of the Mid Markets Bond Department at Morgan Stanley was that management was definitely interested in downsizing the unit and was encouraging many in the group to find employment elsewhere. It seemed the profitability of the business had been squeezed about as far as could be imagined. Top managers were always talking about transparency. When I heard that some bond salesmen had received severance offers, I encouraged Roger Crandal (manager of Institutional Sales for our department) to make me a proposal, emphasizing the retirement factor over severance. By then, I had either told him of my PD affliction or he had deduced its existence by himself. And so in June of 1999, I received a letter that included a satisfactory severance/retirement package. At the age of sixty-one, I weighed the package against my ability to produce commission revenues in a competitive work climate, somewhat softened by the relationships I had developed, in an atmosphere of deteriorating physical capability caused by my PD. As I contemplated my future, I envisioned perhaps just a few more years of golf and good times of traveling. After considering Morgan Stanley's offer for about two or three days, I decided to retire. My date was set for July 1, 1999, which meant my career officially spanned from January 3, 1963 to that date, or 36.5 years.

In slightly more than two years, history totally vindicated my decision. If I had continued working at Morgan Stanley, I would have been directly entangled in the terrorist acts associated with September 11, 2001.

Early in 1999, Morgan Stanley had pulled regional sales personnel from their outposts in the suburbs into the World Trade Center. In my own case, I made the move from the Short Hills office (which was located just five minutes from my home in Chatham) to the twin tower complex. The Mid Markets Group soon took up the space vacated by the institutional equities group and we were quite visible on the trading desk at the sixtieth floor of the WTC #2. Access to the floor required changing elevator banks at the forty-fourth floor, which was referred to as the Sky Plaza.

On that fateful day, I was working on my home computer with my personal computer whiz Bob Van Hook. When I saw the American Airlines jet crash into WTC #2, I could almost feel the impact some twenty-three miles away. The plane seemed to accomplish a direct hit on my former desk. Although almost all (if not all) of my coworkers from that department survived, I am not sure how I would have done given my PD handicap. According to witnesses on the sixtieth floor, Bryan was a true hero in getting the troops to hit the stairways immediately after the first jet hit WTC #1. I am confident Bryan would have made sure of my safety and I would have followed Bryan's example. But perhaps I would have been asleep in the bathroom!

My Parkinson's disease particularly impacted my relationship with one of my best accounts, and didn't exactly revolve around being able to "rock and roll" in the trading markets. One of my original clients, in 1964, was the Raritan Savings Bank in Raritan, New Jersey. Arlyn Rus was the president and CEO of the bank and Charles Smith was its executive VP. Both executives were relatively young and Charlie would have to wait

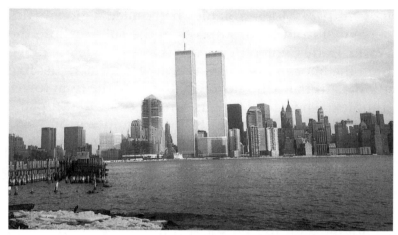

The World Trade Center and the skyline of New York City, circa 1985. Prior to terrorist acts of 2001, the WTC's main occupant was Dean Witter & Company, and subsequently Morgan Stanley, Inc.
(Photo credit: Paul Luscombe)

an eternity for Arlyn to retire so he could advance at the Raritan.

In the late 1960s, the Raritan and many of the other New Jersey mutual savings banks were active bond market participants. Charlie ran the portfolio after he wrestled it away from the crusty Lou Mack of the advisory firm of Beck, Mack & Oliver. As the period came to a close, and as the bond market turned sharply south, Charlie was left with only one position from our trading antics—Duke Power 8⅛ percent First Mortgage Bonds, due in 2007. In the high interest rate cycle that followed, Charlie rode those bonds all the way from 102 to 60. A $1 million piece of the bonds saw its market value decline from $1.02 millionto $600,000. Charlie was miffed that he had one issue classified at such a loss. Many of Charlie's peers had several such holdings that jeopardized their very existence.

In 1983, the tiny Keene Savings Bank (NH) was barely surviving this high interest rate cycle. Rates on U.S. Treasuries (at 15%) caused huge outflows (dubbed "dis-intermediation") at the nation's thrift institutions. Somehow, the Keene Bank contacted Charlie Smith to offer him the top spot at their bank in hopes he could save the franchise. To the surprise of most of the New Jersey banking community, Charlie took the job in New Hampshire. Although I had no other accounts in New Hampshire, Charlie insisted that I cover his new affiliation in the banking world.

Charlie immediately set out to advance the stature of Keene Savings. He saturated the town of Keene with ATMs. He reduced staff. He shortened the bond portfolio. He eventually demutualized the bank and created stock ownership in the institution. And he created the Keene Savings Bank economic seminar, the original guest speaker being one Paul Luscombe. We had a lot to talk about then. The fragile status of the nation's financial markets was on everyone's mind. The local press, led by the *Keene Sentinel*, gave me a good review, the local businessmen peppered me with questions, and most of all, Charley enjoyed the speech. For the next thirteen years, I would mount the podium in Keene and deliver a thirty-minute speech on the economy, the stock market, and the political scene. I would always wind up the talk with a forecast of the level of the U.S. Treasury long bond. My remarks were pitted against John Tuccillo's, who joined the speaker rostrum about 1991. As the economist for the National Association of Homebuilders, John was a "real" economist and had a Ph.D. in the field. My doctorate of Bondology was not listed on my resume.

During these years, this speech was a very important challenge to me. Never did I get up on the stage in Keene and just wing it! I spent many hours researching the markets, reading all the periodicals possible, and I tried to evolve a meaningful overview of the economy that differed from the standard outlook coming out of most brokerage firms. The local businessmen seemed to respect our ideas and I believe they were awed by our ability to accurately forecast long-term interest rates.

On seven separate occasions, I gave the Keene Economic Address knowing I was afflicted with Parkinson's. As my condition worsened, however gradually, I began to contemplate the possibility of starting to tremble in the middle of my talk or having some other physical breakdown. I didn't want to disappoint Charley, but these fears kept me awake for nights on end. Finally, I decided to tell Charley about my affliction. Some several months before the talk, I wrote him a long letter and followed up with a phone call. It was one of the most difficult decisions I made in my life. I was retiring from the Keene Economic Seminar for health reasons.

Even though I had resigned as guest speaker, Charley and the bank always invited me to subsequent seminars. Charley also salved my ego a bit by introducing me as the "retired lecturer" at subsequent seminars.

Through a series of mergers, Keene Savings Bank changed its name to the Granite Bank of Keene (NH), and by 2003 it had become the largest independent bank in the state of New Hampshire. The Chittenden Trust Co of Burlington, Vermont made a merger proposal to Charley and soon the bank was gone as an autonomous entity. The Chittenden bank opted to discontinue the economic seminar. To all of us involved, it was the end of an era.

On the subject of public speaking—I have had several occasions to appear before large groups, since I discovered I have Parkinson's. At the time of some of these speeches I was in the preliminary phases of Parkinson's disease. For ten years, I ran the Hall of Fame for Lafayette College in Easton, Pennsylvania. The position entailed being the emcee at the organization's annual induction dinner. Conceptually, the HOF remarks were less strenuous than speaking about the economy, but still the specter of trembling or losing voice power led me to quit the HOF position. Anyway, I felt that ten years was way too long for a chairman to have sway over the committee. Regardless, I was proud of the selections made during my tenure. I thought my idea of Lafayette College Athletes of the Century to celebrate the year 2000 was particularly successful. Although a time consuming effort, I enjoyed reuniting some of the successful teams from Lafayette's history, even though the effort was criticized for lengthening the induction dinner ceremony. I think some of the heavy donors to the college complained about the dinner winding up at ten-thirty p.m. At any rate, after ten years—Parkinson's or no Parkinson's—it was time for someone else to take over. A Hall of Fame requires that the selections be as objective as possible. A rotating chairmanship should at least contribute to that ideal.

Before being diagnosed with Parkinson's, I had envisioned doing part-time work in the securities business. I also thought I could obtain a limited position in the Alumni Relations department of Lafayette College. The problem with my version of Parkinson's is simply that I cannot drive a car anywhere. As the disease has worsened, I have even less mobility, needing a walker (or rollader) or wheelchair to get around. From time to time, I had a lot of driving support and this helped me deliver the books written for PAL Publishing.

From a therapeutic standpoint, in no way did I foresee the advantages of the PAL phenomenon. With very limited deadlines, the self-publishing company gave me a ton of freedom. I had no grumpy old editors telling me what to do or write. Once the VBK book (*Play the Game Right)* was under way, I had a full-time project on my hands. Ultimately, the Howard book (*Howard Powerless)* required the same amount of energy. Although I sought a publisher with a national distribution system, I wonder if I could have been effective under "foreign management."

While in retirement, I have retained my membership in two professional societies—the Bond Club of New Jersey and the Money Marketeers of New York University. In the case of the BCNJ, I only just recently resigned from the organization's board of governors. I served almost six years on the board as a retiree, and although I found the position stimulating, I also gradually started to lose touch with trends in the industry. It is probably a fine distinction, but I enjoyed the organization as a means of cementing relationship business. Clients and competitors all mixed together at golf outings and social events like A Night at the Races. But as the merger movement reduced the number of independent institutions in New Jersey, the organization transformed into more of a networking organization.

Dealers, brokers, bond fund representatives, and branch managers from such firms as Morgan Stanley and Wachovia Securities were the main participants. I worked very hard to recruit members who fit the relationship profile but who were not part of the networking lineup per se. Most of my recent member proposals have enjoyed an outing or two, but then suddenly were heard from no more.

The Money Marketeers is less of a social organization and more of a forum for prominent public speakers from the arena of economics, the Federal Reserve System, and occasionally the Department of the Treasury. We have also heard some leading Central Bankers of major foreign countries. My father belonged to the organization in the 1940s, and I am sure he learned a lot about the operation of the money and capital markets from Marcus Nadler, the founder of the club. The club is a little bit difficult for me to use because all its events are in New York City. I am working with the leadership of the club right now in hopes they will highlight my *Howard Powerless* books at one of the club's future forums.

I sometimes wonder if my many years (almost thirty-seven) on Wall Street and stress on my mental and physical faculties had anything to do with my contracting Parkinson's disease. A major change in my career path occurred in 1984, when I elected to move from my original employer (Halsey Stuart & Co, subsequently renamed Bache Halsey Stuart Shields Inc) to Alex. Brown & Sons, which claimed to be the oldest investment bank in the United States. Steve Barrett, the partner in charge of the corporate bond department, was the catalyst for the move. At the age of forty-six, I was ready for a change. A series of liquid lunches with Steve at the Wall Street restaurant known as Captain's Ketch led me to the point where I shook hands and said yes.

Actually, the turmoil at my soon to be former employer was quite intense. The new team at Bache basically resembled the former players for AG Becker, and many of us on the "A" Bache team were unhappy with the way Becker moved in and unceremoniously replaced or downgraded "our guys."

Bache salesmen were continuously pulled off their accounts in favor of Becker representatives. I knew I faced a battle with former Becker salesman Jimmy Hall over the First Fidelity account. Becker was known for its block trading in stocks and bonds, Bache had a retail mentality, and I felt a degree of insecurity in this environment. As I went to work every day in this unhappy work climate, I was constantly reminded of the soothing message of Steve Barrett at Alex Brown. Steve offered me all my existing accounts plus any others I could bring on board. Joe Colleran—one of the first to leave the Bache-Becker combo—was one of my best friends in the business and he was firmly in place at Brown as the long utility trader. Joe gave me a first-hand, "thumbs up" report on ABSB and soon I was ready to make my first job change ever.

I should have hurried back from lunch the day I shook hands with Steve and walked into Bob Kelly's office and said, "I am quitting." Instead, I left Steve with the assurance that I would tell my Bache/Becker boss by the end of the week. For three nights, I couldn't sleep as I wondered how my boss would react, what my coworkers would think—a ton of negative thoughts crossed my mind. I had come to Halsey Stuart right out of college and worked there and for successor firms for more than twenty years. For three days, I could hardly look anyone in the eye as I focused on doing my months' old expense accounts. Herb Mathiasen, who kept track of such matters, said that was a dead giveaway that someone was about to leave the firm. Others commented on the neatness of my normally cluttered desk!

On Friday, October 23, 1984, I finally stood outside Bob Kelly's office waiting for him to get off the phone. I was joined in the foyer by John Griff, a prominent syndicate department player who also had a resignation speech prepared. John entered Kelly's office before me and quietly made his case to our mutual boss. Kelly seemed upset at the loss of John Griff, a rising star in the corporate bond competitive bidding wars. In-house, we nicknamed John "The Unguided Missile" in recognition of his buying a Beckton Dickinson corporate note issue from the company just minutes before the Federal Reserve Bank cut the discount rate.

While Kelly tried to digest Griff's resignation, I stepped into his office, butterflies in my stomach, listening to his disappointment with "The Missile's" departure. When he finished telling me about Griff, he seemed totally unprepared for my statement. Unbeknownst to me, I was slated to be one of the veteran salesmen of the new Becker-Bache team. Apparently my role was somewhat significant. I told him of my opportunity at Alex Brown and my desire to make a change before I hit fifty years old. But Kelly just wouldn't let go, and soon he summoned Ed Ellingham, one of my lifelong friends and Kelly's number two man, into his office to try and prevail upon me to stay at Becker-Bache. Never an alarmist, Ed was compassionate and asked if Steve and I did in fact shake hands. I assured him that Steve Barrett and I had a meeting of the minds and that I was intent on making the move. Ed convinced me to rethink the offer over the weekend, which only prolonged the agony of finally severing the chord with Bache. On Monday morning, I came into 100 Gold Street for my final day of work and told management that I was leaving the firm.

In this world of multiple divorces and free agent sports figures, it probably doesn't seem that a simple job change would cause much stress. Believe me, I made my vodka martinis a lot stronger during this entire episode. Soon, I would have to prove myself to my new employer, then a partnership, Alex Brown & Sons.

I started immediately at Alex Brown, and soon I launched the most successful and happiest leg of my entire business career. My ability to do business was instantaneous! On my very first day, while Steve Barrett was introducing me to my new team of coworkers, a phone call came in looking for me on the trading floor. Within full view of the entire department, I received an order from Charlie Smith in New Hampshire to buy 5,000 shares of ATT common stock. The block stock trader Peter Irish (also a friend from Chatham) quickly handled the trade, and before I could say Paul Volcker, I was on the books at Alex Brown. I will be forever grateful to Charley Smith for my grand entrance.

My other clients quickly fell in line, as I seemed to have my own customized trading desk. Soon Kevin McCardle was on board from the old Bache "A" team. Then came my former sales manager, Bruce Yeutter. The flow of business was marvelous! The Alex Brown management let me highlight the nation by allowing me to call on corporations for the purpose of acquiring their own debt in the market place. They encouraged creativity, and I remember trading bonds with General Telephone Company of California. The monetary rewards followed—I probably was the top corporate bond salesman for 1985 and 1986. Also, I participated in the firm's initial public offering of common stock. I was suddenly a very happy and modestly wealthy bond salesman.

But this was the 1980s and unprecedented volatility prevailed in all sectors of the stock and bond markets. As the prime rate soared to over 20 percent in the mid 1980s, bond prices plunged to historically low levels. As Steve Barret attempted to build the department, some of his forays into longer dated telephone and utility bonds resulted in massive trading losses. Although the new Alex Brown corporate trading team was very profitable, the guttural communication style over the firm's loud speaker (known on Wall Street as the Hoot & Holler) seemed to negatively affect the staid old management types in Baltimore. Management suddenly was meeting behind closed doors and considering a new business plan, apparently with an exclusive dedication to the junk bond market.

On Monday, October 19, 1987, the Dow Jones Industrial Average lost 22 percent of its value, marking the largest single-day decline in the history of the stock market. On the following day, Tuesday, October 20, Steve Barrett summoned the entire corporate bond department into a meeting. With little buildup, he bluntly explained that the company of Alex Brown & Sons was closing the corporate bond department as we knew it and would continue on as a specialized junk bond operation. Quietly and a bit subtly, I had just been fired.

I just couldn't believe what had happened. When I returned to my desk, I noticed the Washington Savings Bank had called looking for some bids. When I approached Kevin McCardle for some indications, he replied: "You asshole! Weren't you listening? We are closed!"

It had to be one of the major shocks of my life! I loved my job, I loved my coworkers, and I was making money in the process. Now I would have to hop on the interview trail and try to find a comparable position within the industry. Once the word spread, the phone calls seeking my services started to roll in! One of the very first calls was from Joe Colleran, who had jumped to Dean Witter & Co. at the World Trade Center Tower #2. Before noon, Joe had set me up with my first interview, lunch the following day with Ed Ellinigham, who had come over from the former Becker-Bache team months earlier. When I toured the DW trading floor on the sixtieth floor of the WTC #2, it sure had the appearance of the AG Becker unit that had been in command at Bache Halsey when I left in 1984. The head of taxable fixed income was none other than Bob Kelly, the man to whom I submitted my resignation.

My initial days at Dean Witter in no way resembled my start at Alex Brown & Sons. I soon discovered that the company was deep in an internal struggle as it tried to reconcile the objectives of the institutional and retail departments. The Sears ownership seemed to favor the retail side of the business, and often acted to inhibit the style of the institutional effort. Before I wrote my first ticket at Dean Witter, rumors were flying that the corporate bond department serving institutions would soon be closed, and the specter of massive layoffs loomed everywhere on the sixtieth floor.

I found no benefit in listening to these rumors. I decided to try and establish a business niche within this limited quasi retail-institutional framework. The commission payout on retail business was substantially higher than institutional trades, and therefore I only needed to do half the business just to remain at my same net production level. I basically had one trader—Mike Papa—who could handle my order flow. As the institutional department evaporated, the retail management team that prevailed was impressed with our level of business. Soon the head of the retail bond department for taxable fixed income—Bob Dwyer—invited me and Mike to join his team. Mike was indeed a clever and imaginative trader. He knew his markets, he respected his intermediary street brokers, and he kept me constantly abreast of interesting opportunities in the market. Over my thirty-seven years on Wall Street, Mike was easily one of the best traders I ever worked with. Soon Bob restocked the corporate trading desk and Mike and I were considered charter members of the group. It was a most unusual ride requiring a lot of hard work and pressure, but Mike and I felt good about our modest success. In the process of our operations, Bryan was rehired by the Dwyer team.

In 1988, as I turned fifty years old, I was adopting a new style of doing business. I could feel the stress of my efforts. I constantly entertained the young members of my corporate team on Thursday evenings in New York City. I still remember some vigorous but friendly arguments with Brian Colleran (Joe's younger brother) about who was the

Man of the Century. I was forever supportive of Gorbachev, while Brian favored Dwight Eisenhower.

Dean Witter transformed into a good place to be in the early 1990s. About the same time that I was diagnosed with PD, Chairman Phil Purcell and President Jim Higgins took the firm public, and I was a ready participant. During the next seven years, I accumulated a fair amount of DWD stock (and subsequently Morgan Stanley stock). On several occasions, I also earned a slot in the President's Club (representing the firm's top 10% in production), which entailed some trips to the likes of Palm Beach, Florida and Palm Springs, California. Working with Bryan was a joy! Working on Wall Street could be fun after all!

I feel the bizarre events of my voluntary job departure from Bache Halsey Stuart and my involuntary exit from Alex Brown plus the turmoil I initially experienced at Dean Witter may have worked some havoc on my brain. Although I probably showed little if any outward signs of stress, perhaps I subliminally felt the pressure stronger than I thought.

Simultaneous with the ebb and flow of forces at my job, I had to deal with a rather traumatic experience on the home front. For years, my wife and I had been planning to enlarge the size of our house at 44 Dunbar Street in Chatham. We initially moved to this house in 1967, and our plans to build a den on the side of the house were ruled by the Borough Planning Committee to be too close to our property line. Variances were given to many property owners in Chatham, but for some reason our efforts were thwarted by the planning committee.

In the winter of 1988, the Bilhubers decided to sell their relatively large house located just two blocks from our Dunbar Street home. You could look out our kitchen window and see the Bilhuber residence on Carmine Street. It seemed like an easy decision to sell our house and buy the Bilhubers' house and have the additions we wanted already in place. It was like a value added bond trade, and I assured my somewhat hesitant wife that we had to move quickly in order to snag the Bilhuber house before other ready buyers did. It was one of the largest houses in the area, and sat on a substantial double lot. We purchased the house for $425,000 in a private transaction.

I soon discovered it was easier to move a $425,000 piece of bonds than it was to execute a real estate transaction. Several incidents marred the closing. For example, subsequent to our signing the purchase contract, they installed a sump pump in the basement. With Chatham being a low lying area, a sump pump was a necessity for those homes prone to flooding. We had no sump pump on Dunbar Street and our original walk-through showed no such device on Carmine either. Skepticism and doubt prevailed throughout the period between contract and closing. The day of the closing saw the movers arrive at our house at eight a.m. and finish up more than twelve hours later. I thought the day would never end!

We soon started adjusting to our new home. In the course of my activities, I had reason to venture to the basement, probably to fetch another type of screwdriver than the one I had removed from my workbench. As I went to grab the railing that I thought was on the lefthand side of the stairway (as was the case in our Dunbar Street home), I suddenly was grasping nothing but air and I took a hard fall down the steps, spinning as I tried to brace my fall, and landing virtually with my back impaled on top of Bilhuber's sump pump.

My back never really recovered from the fall. For years, I was treated by a local chiropractor and basketball teammate, Gerry Milazzo. Dr. Gardner in Morristown finally performed a disc operation on my back. I also tried a minimally invasive back operation with Dr. Knightly of Chatham. The 1990–2000 era was great for business, but caused me all sorts of pain physically.

The fall when I hurt my back occurred in 1988. I was diagnosed with PD in 1992. Prior to the fall, I had little or no problem with my back. Nor did I experience the Parkinson's symptoms beforehand. Nowhere, to my knowledge, is there any history of PD in my family. In my own mind, I link this hard fall with my Parkinson's problem.

My favorite extracurricular activity in the 1980s was playing basketball in the Chatham Men's Basketball League. Prior to 1980, the town had open gym sessions in the high school on Wednesday evenings and Sunday afternoons. The court time was intended for the use of Chatham residents and those who worked in the town. But with virtually no control device in hand, the games got quite unwieldy as players—virtually teams—from outside the area made the trip to play in Chatham. What began as a friendly Sunday afternoon exercise session soon evolved into rough competitive basketball. The crowds grew to the point that unless you were on one of the stronger teams known to be winners, you played one quick game of ten points and you were done for the day. The core of legitimate Chatham players was indeed upset with the whole arrangement.

After a few years of experimenting with a league structure, I created a league that was more driven by social groups within the Chatham framework. For example, the

Chatham Jaycees fielded a team, as did the Chatham Newcomers Club. A fifteen-dollar registration fee entitled the player to an official league t-shirt and assured him of a slot on one of the seven teams. Whenever a new family moved into town, I was there to recruit the adult male for the league. We played every Wednesday and Sunday between December 1 and March 31, concluding the season with a round-robin tourney. I published the league standings and leading scorers in the local newspaper. We kept the league going with a lenient rule on forfeits—four on four counted as an actual league game, for example. And if a team needed an extra player to fill the four-man minimum, I availed my talents so that a forfeit could be avoided. Some nights I played in two games, and I was pretty wiped out by the time things wrapped up.

I became known in town as the Commissioner of Basketball. Early on, in 1983, the players gave me a plaque recognizing my efforts. Then, in 1989, they gave me a pewter mug that said, "The Commissioner". The town Board of Recreation gave me a plaque that same year as a part its annual Spirit Award program.

Upon turning fifty, my ability to compete actively in the Chatham Men's League started to wear thin. Also, NFL football player Neil O'Donnell became a legitimate roster member when his brother Steve moved into the Southern Passaic Avenue apartments near the train station. Neil was completing his senior year at Maryland University when Steve moved into town and almost immediately made application to be the eighth team in the Chatham Men's League. Their nickname was the Fightin' Irish, and they immediately stormed through the schedule undefeated. They didn't play for exercise and enjoyment . . . they actually played to win!

My colleagues from the League insisted on a special meeting; the intensity of the Irish as well as some of their alleged ringers was the topic of discussion. I visited Steve O'Donnell at his nearby apartment and tried to get him to calm down his players, mostly members of his own family!

We couldn't expel the Irish for winning, and so I resigned as the "commissioner." My back, which suffered from the fall down the stairs in our new house, made it very difficult for me to play anyway. My final game was against the Irish and I guarded Neil O'Donnell. Neil outscored me 44–4.

One of the highlights of my basketball interest was my selection by the Chatham Jaycees to play in their annual fundraiser basketball game against the New York Giants. My standing on the team was honorary and in no way related to my ability to play. At age fifty, I was easily the oldest player on the court.

After going through the motions of a lay-up drill, I sat down on the bench and watched the game. The Giants literally toyed with the best players that the Jaycees could recruit (i.e., Jim Liccardo, Colt Heppe, and Dan McHale), and the first quarter went by quickly. Then I heard Mo Ryan of the Jaycees call my name, and I was in the game. The court was quite a bit longer than I was used to, and I quickly tired as I tried to keep up with the physically superior Giants. My responsibility was to guard Carl Banks, then an outstanding linebacker in the NFL. A minute or two passed, and we were on offense when I set a pick for Jim Liccardo, our best shooter. While the ball was in the air, I rolled toward the basket in hopes of getting the rebound. But Banks had me completely boxed out, and he soared to surely snare the re-

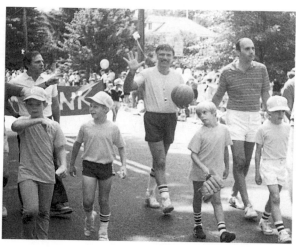

The commissioner of basketball for Chatham Borough (with ball) marches in the 4th of July Parade in 1985. Former Duke University star and the League's high scorer, Jim Liccardi, marches alongside Luscombe.
(Photo credit: Cinnie Luscombe)

bound. However, Liccardo's shot was very soft and teetered on the rim. Banks had committed to his leap too soon, and I started my ascent as he was on the way down. I soon had a free tap in and put the ball through the hoop! I was no longer "honorary"! I was on the score pad! My small throng of fans gave me a rousing cheer!

During the second half, I again sat on the bench until late in the game. I didn't realize it, but my minimal playing time in the first half, then sitting for almost an hour, caused me to stiffen up considerably. Once back in the game, I felt my back give in and I was sure happy when the game was over. The incident, though fun to brag about, was no fun as far as my back was concerned. This tough game coupled with falling down the stairs at our new house on Carmine Street, led me to have back and sciatic problems thereafter.

When I first knew that I was affected by Parkinson's disease, I used to cover up my condition by saying that I probably played too many years of basketball. Perhaps it had some influence on my walking later in life. All the while, I thought I was doing something that was good for me!

Post retirement, my original business card read "Private Investor", which gave me a marginal identity. When I created PAL Publishing, my business card changed to read "President". A very proud identity, indeed!

Chapter 5B

The PAL Publishing Company

The PAL Publishing Company was founded in 2000. Tireless efforts to convince known publishers to put my material in print produced no results. My wife gave me a directory of publishers of all sizes and locations, and we must have called each and every one of them. We also unsuccessfully combed the Yellow Pages of all of New York and New Jersey. I even took leads given to me from John Feinstein, who was the guest speaker at a Lafayette College dinner where I was the emcee. As one of America's top sports novelists (*A Good Walk Spoiled, The Last Amateurs, Season on the Brink, The Punch,* etc.), he gave me contacts at Random House, Simon & Schuster, and Little Brown & Co., but none would underwrite my story on Butch van Breda Kolff.

And so I took steps to become a self-publisher. I registered myself as a business operating in New Jersey and bought a strip consisting of ten International Standard Book Numbers for $250. Known as ISBNs, these numbers officially record that the book is copy-written material. I then opened up a bank account at the local branch of the Peapack Gladstone Bank. Now more than four years later, Parkinson's notwithstanding, I have written four books and distributed close to 2,300 copies.

To date, there are no shares of PAL Publishing outstanding. I am the self-appointed chief executive officer and function as the company's president. The company has been set up as a sole proprietorship. Friends like Doug Hobby, Raymond Monroe, Kelly Dotson, and Ken Thompson assist me in mailing operations, driving responsibilities, and other distribution functions. You will note that this is the same group referred to as the Chatham Mens Club in a previous chapter. Likewise, these four friends were great in helping me recover from my appendicitis attack in February 2004.

To my wife's chagrin, the PAL Publishing Company is headquartered in the living room of our home in Chatham. After confronting our twelve-year-old blind Pekinese (named Gizmo), the first item one sees is a card table laden with copies of my three already published books and manuscripts from the book I am trying to assemble. Soda and water bottles, snacks and leftover dishes are strewn between the various writings. Try as I may, it seems impossible to keep the area neat.

In addition to my responsibilities as chief executive officer of PAL activities, I must manage and monitor the family nest-egg, which is basically a portfolio of stocks and bonds, including some hybrid securities such as preferred stocks and convertible bonds.

My objective is to generate income sufficient to support my family's living expenses. Hopefully, the stocks will provide a modicum of growth that will offset any invasion of principle. The portfolio is anything but passive, and I am constantly seeking opportunities to enhance performance. Complicating the whole process has been the implementation of some sort of tax strategy. About 21 percent of the funds are professionally managed by Keating Investment Counselors of Del Ray Beach, Florida. With one exception, Keating is fully invested in pure equity holdings.

My income derived from operating PAL Publishing is quite modest; to date around $10,000. Since the birth of PAL, I have tended to retain most all of the earnings and have plowed them back into the production of yet another book.

Related to my PAL Publishing activity is my role as an officer of the Class of 1960 at Lafayette College. Since graduating some forty-five years ago, I have been the class correspondent and have published several articles per year in the school's publication entitled *The Lafayette Alumni News*. Twice I have received awards as the Correspondent of the Year. Over the years, the column has given me great satisfaction, and judging by the comments of my classmates, has been well received on their part as well. Otherwise, they wouldn't have re-elected me nine times! I also try to organize a Class of 1960 golf outing sometime every summer.

Additionally, at the organization's request, until recently, I served on the board of governors of the Bond Club of New Jersey as one of their leaders. My time for running outings and administering the Club took place in the mid 1970s.The Club used my experience in setting up its annual meeting, constructing its membership directory, and taking care of a host of other affairs.

Writing the books and LC articles, running the miniature company, managing the family investments, helping out the BCNJ, playing a little golf, and attending various sporting events kept me extremely busy and helped me forget about my own personal health problems.

The tricky part of the whole program was managing to accomplish most of my objectives during the on time of my PD. Very little can be accomplished in the off times.

Most of my prolific writing comes in the very early morning. I frequently think of a creative writing idea while in my sleep or when I'm about to wake up, and so I try to get to work as soon as possible. I usually can write for about two hours (from six to eight a.m.) before I have to get to some other activities such as walking the dog and lining up my wife's morning coffee. Since I do sit so long, it is absolutely critical that I periodically get up and stretch my legs a bit. Of course there is a well-worn path to the refrigerator!

One problem I have is that my hands consistently stick to the keys on my computer keyboard or mouse; thus my ability to touch type is somewhat compromised. I can type much faster and create more fluidly if I don't have to keep watching the screen at all times. However, the muscular restraint I feel, particularly as I approach an off portion of my cycle, inhibits my ability to produce more finished manuscript in a given period of time. The by-word of any business is "productivity," and PD definitely limits the productivity of the PAL Publishing Company. When the book is in production (i.e., about ready to roll off the printing press), more conversation via telephone is required with the self-publishing printing company I work with in Ohio. Two of my books have been published via BookMasters, Inc. of Mansfield, Ohio. One of the most critical functions for the author is to accurately study and edit the proofs or galleys generated at the printers. This is often difficult for me as a Parkinsonian because the slightest bit of boredom or repetitiveness puts me to sleep. Also, forgetfulness can impact the quality of the book. Sometimes I tend to repeat the same story, perhaps in a different light.

Still, the satisfaction derived from writing and publishing a book is worth the effort. When the UPS driver delivers the first box of 100 hardbound copies of my book to the door, I get a warm and fuzzy feeling, probably symbolizing a sense of real accomplishment. Soon, however, reality sets in. My wife doesn't want to look at 100 (or more) copies of my latest book under the card table in the living room! In fact, if it weren't for Book-Masters' warehouse, my entire first floor would be occupied by my unsold book inventory.

Selling the books on a sustained basis becomes a real challenge once the initial burst of buying takes place. Prior to publication, I spend a substantial amount of time writing letters, making phone calls, utilizing my page on the Internet, and actually visiting some bookstores to seek out demand for my books. My contacts from Lafayette College, the business world, and my friends from Chatham all have been supportive of my writing efforts.

The VBK book—*Play the Game Right: The Biography of Butch van Breda Kolff*—sold out relatively quickly. The opening thrust of sales came at the Lafayette Hall of Fame Dinner when Butch was inducted into the College's elite group. My older daughter Alison and her future husband Erik were active in selling the book after the dinner at the College Hill Tavern. Bob Twimble, then owner of the CHT, kept posters advertising the book prominently on display in the tavern. Posters showing Butch's face were posted at several locations around campus. Bob also helped publicize the VBK book by auctioning several copies at his mid-summer golf outing. My charisma helped me push first day sales to about 100.

The stereotypical author can be seen at most bookstores, publicizing his latest publication and signing his name to the satisfaction of his readers. The effectiveness of this sales technique is limited for the author with PD, however. Autographing a book with an illegible signature is tantamount to damaging the book, and the buyer might insist on a new copy. Most of my autograph sessions are done at a casual pace in the comfort of my home.

I thoroughly underestimated the response to the VBK book, and probably will regret limiting production to only 500 copies. Although a physical challenge, book signings at Princeton University and Lafayette College basketball games added to the momentum. A modest overflow of orders has forced me to turn away business, which tends to show some signs of life during the Big Dance known as the NCAA tourney. In many ways, Butch typified March Madness before the term ever became popular.

My heart went out to Butch van Breda Kolff at a Princeton basketball game versus Dartmouth. An eight-year-old boy, undoubtedly prompted by his father, approached Butch and asked him to autograph his program for the evening. Butch readily obliged, but it took him forever to write out the full four names that make up his full name. Later, I encouraged Butch to simply sign "VBK", but he would have nothing to do with that easy solution. Butch was also a victim of Parkinson's disease.

The Howard Savings Bank book is quite a bit more serious in its content and probably most of the copies have been sold inside the borders of New Jersey. Although the lessons learned are appropriate for all walks of business, the title and emphasis makes the book a bit provincial.

But after a long spell with no book inventory, I decided to publish 800 copies of the Howard book. As I approached the half-sold mark, one of my buyers became quite interested in its content. John Kraft (generally referred to as "Jack"), a fellow member of the Bond Club of New Jersey and a prominent municipal bond attorney, read the book and was captivated by its contents. Jack then took it upon himself to write a review of the book and soon it was reprinted in the *New Jersey Banker* magazine. Immediately, I noticed an improvement in the level of sales. In fact, shortly thereafter, as I was leaving a local New Jersey restaurant, one of the bankers who had bought a book earlier ran up to me and wanted to buy four more books! How could he get them?! We moved to the trunk of my car, where I usually keep a "traveling inventory," and I consummated a four-for-$100 cash deal in the parking lot.

Jack Kraft's efforts didn't stop with the *New Jersey Banker* magazine. Soon, he was working on the *Star Ledger*. Later on, the review appeared in the *New Jersey Law Review*. He even recommended the book as a method of enhancing the business curriculum at Rutgers University's School of Business and wrote the dean in support of his idea.

I had planned on a publicity stunt whereby I set up a booth in front of the local Wachovia branch. Several years ago, the building was the prominent local Howard branch, but was converted to a First Fidelity office when the Howard failed. The local branch manager for WB turned me down, however. Perhaps they didn't want any recalcitrant stockholders identifying them with the Howard name.

At one point in time, the Howard listed more than 1,000 employees, and I was determined to at least inform a large portion of these workers about the book. Somehow, former investment officers John Quinn and Susan Penona arrived on the scene with a list of close to 500 ex-employees.

They represented a group of potential returnees for a Howard Savings reunion. The chore of single-handedly culling through the 500 names seemed overwhelming, and so I got an estimate of what it would cost to have a letter printed and envelopes addressed and mailed. The cost seemed prohibitive, and so I decided to tackle the project all on my own. Parkinson Paul then proceeded to write out close to 300 envelopes. I thought that the list might contain some obsolete addresses. But rather than using that as an excuse, I decided to go ahead. As I started out writing fairly slowly, the first few addresses didn't look too bad, but with each passing envelope, my handwriting grew more and more illegible. Some envelopes had quite large lettering, some had small, almost cryptic letters. Growing exhausted and more and more frustrated, I called my friend Doug Hobby to help me complete the project.

Doug has no known physical problems and his handwriting is quite legible. He wrote about 200 of the envelopes and I was cut off at my 300 level. Doug literally commandeered the mailroom of PAL Publishing! Following the coup, Doug delegated me to folding letters, applying stamps, and other less cosmetic functions. During the project, we humorously answered the telephone with a loud and cheerful "Mailroom!" I fixed Doug one of his patented Perfect Bourbon Manhattan's in order to keep him in a good mood!

The immediate response to the mail project was a deluge of letters marked with a yellow sticker "RTS/ return to sender". Illegible names and addresses were the main source of the returns, although the official reasons listed on the envelope included: (1) insufficient address (2) attempted not known (3) no such number or street, and (4) not deliverable as addressed. More than fifty envelopes were returned. As I quickly eyeballed the returned letters, I could tell that almost all of them were mine. Only a handful were from Doug's section, and those were probably due to the person moving to another location. (See an example of my envelope below.)

PAL Publishing & Co.
C/o Paul A Luscombe, Pres.
8 Carmine Street,
Chat m, NJ 07928

At first, I was mad at myself for wasting so much time and effort. But Doug pointed out that at least 250 or so of mine made it to their proper destination. The more I thought about it, I guess I did pretty well after all.

In the aftermath, my friend Raymond Monroe and his pal Kelly Dodson collected all the returned envelopes and rewrote them to be more legible and deliverable. The chore was easily accomplished in an hour or so.

Imperfection. You can list it as just another of the many Perils of Parkinson's Disease.

You never know where you will find a prolific sales outlet. I must have a friend in the owner of Schnippers Gift & Stationary store in Madison, New Jersey. Tony Pross has probably sold more copies of my books than the local bookstore has in Chatham! He likes to stress the local nature of my books and he likes to dwell on the fact the book is autographed. He retains a stack of my books, when appropriate, right at the cash register. I give Doug Hobby the credit for discovering Schnippers during our attempt to market the Mulligan Book at local country clubs!

Another hang-up of the Parkinson's Publisher is that of meeting deadlines. In the case of the Howard book, my intended publication date was July 2003. I wrote letters to my loyal core of readers and solicited checks, telling recipients of this July date, just in time for many to read during the summer months. However, just when I was getting busy with other activities, I discovered I needed to make a few changes in basic content late in the production cycle, which caused me to rewrite two entire chapters. My off cycles weren't doing me any favors either, and so the book came to market in mid November 2003.

Ed Bantlow is a classmate of mine from Lafayette College. By profession, I would classify him as an entrepreneur. He received his MBA from Harvard and seems to be involved with many different businesses. Ed was always admonishing me to write about broader topics or personalities. His preference over VBK would have been Shaquille O'Neal, and so on down the line. Others at Lafayette encouraged me to write the biography of Arthur Rothkopf, the college's outstanding president for eleven or so years. But I preferred to write about topics for which I had a ton of original material. My college basketball program collection from the mid 1950s helped me with some original ideas about VBK. My friendships with Don Kress, Walter Hislop, and John Quinn led me to writing about the Howard.

PAL Publishing Company was strictly a conduit for me to keep busy and hopefully entertain some readers who have interests similar to mine. In many respects, the books gave me a sense of accomplishment. Perhaps, in some circles, I was a mini-celebrity.

Another source of satisfaction or psychic income emanated from the book company. For the summers of 2002 and 2003, I had two sets of interns from Lafayette College working for me. In 2002, Ryan Schaffer and Lauren Frese helped me research the background for the Howard Savings Bank book, and in 2003, Emily Groves and Teril Klein helped me rev up for the sales promotion of the book. My wife set up visits to the *New York Times* and the *Star Ledger,* which enlightened our understanding of how a modern newspaper was produced.

Though respectable in our society, the label "retiree" may imply a way of life that entails little motivation or accomplishment. Post retirement, my original

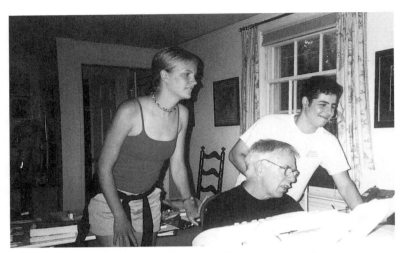

Interns from Lafayette College who helped author Luscombe work on the production of **Howard Powerless** *include Emily Groves and Teril Kline. The student publishers received credit for their curriculum while working for the PAL Publishing Company.*
(Photo credit: Cynthia Luscombe)

business card read *"Private Investor"*, which gave me a marginal identity. When I created PAL Publishing, my business card changed to read *"President"*. A very proud identity, indeed! At the Lafayette Reunion Weekend in June 2004, as you entered the College Bookstore, you were greeted by a prominent display of books authored by various Lafayette alumni. I was quite pleased to see two of my books seated in the first row of the display, and I am sure my ego was inflated just a tad.

Somewhere in the course of my activities as an author, I had the chance to build a Web page to publicize and provide an ordering mechanism for my books. Maria Dragone and Matt Anthony, a very successful sister and brother team specializing in Web hosting and programming, set me up with my Web page, which can be seen on the Internet at www.palpublishing.com. The page has several sections, including synopses of all my books, my personal history, contact information, order forms, and other vital information. The Web team duo are listed under the name Psi Prime Incorporated in West Paterson, New Jersey.

On "cleanup day," my wife takes to the war path—every
light bulb must be changed, every battery must be checked,
and all recycling must be put in the queue. I try to stay
out of the way, and frequently schedule a lunch date.

Chapter 6

The Dreaded Cleanup Day

I must admit that the various activities described broadly in the chapters entitled "Remaining Socially Active" and "The PAL Publishing Company" are accomplished unfortunately with a degree of fallout as far as neatness is concerned. Streams of paperwork drape my desk, with PAL Publishing providing the most significant volume. Experimental manuscripts, correspondence, and mail relating to PAL—all this very valuable paperwork blankets most of two card tables and a large portion of my desk. I also try to keep on display the books I have already published as a reminder to those who drop by that I actually have books for sale.

Each category has its own pile, and I try to keep them all organized and neat, but such is not the forte of the imaginative and creative artist. Often, when driven to clean up my area, all I do is shift the papers from one pile to another. I also may create a new pile and place it in a not so conspicuous location. Hardly anything hits the trash or recycle bin.

Then there are matters pertaining to the management of my family's investment portfolios. We all have separate accounts and separate IRAs, which I monitor with the support of a telephone-book sized notebook containing each monthly statement. Given the Parkinson's disease victim's tendency toward amnesia, I always try to verify my ownership of a particular stock or bond before actually entering a sell order. Also, in March and April, I am inundated with annual reports and proxy materials relating to our broad ownership in common stocks. I also keep records of our various insurance policies, local taxes, medical deductions for tax purposes, and on and on.

In fact, my tax return for the 2004 calendar year provides a real live example of the paperwork involved with my life. My returns for federal and state taxes (both New Jersey and New York) added up to forty-five pages. I also had to save and file away documentation relating to the calculations contained on my returns. Additionally, I helped my daughters gather their tax information for the accountant. Somehow, when my daughter Priscilla's W-2 was missing from her file, I was the one to blame! Goes with the territory, I guess.

I try to separate material relating to Lafayette College. In my forty-fifth year as class correspondent for the Class of 1960, I am always trying to accumulate information on my classmates, and so this becomes an open file. Eventually, this pile gets transferred to the computer to be ultimately written as a story to be published in the Lafayette *Alumni News*. Also, I am the designated class agent, authorized to update the official Class of 1960 page on the Internet. As chairman of the Class of 1960 Golf Tourney, I create yet another significant "pile" of material. I also just completed a category relating to our forty-fifth Reunion in June 2005. Additionally, notices of general alumni social activities, sporting events, fund raisers, and the like are all kept in a special place, most notably the inside cover of my address book. This year, the correspondence pertaining to the naming of a new president to succeed the retiring Arthur Rothkopf was of special interest.

More incoming material flows as a result of my involvement with the Bond Club of NJ. In retirement, I remained on the board of governors for six years. I performed a multitude of duties (recruit members, organize the annual meeting, etc.), which also added to my clutter. I am part of an ad hoc committee of four board members studying the installation of a BCNJ Web site this fall. If finalized, odds are I will be the one to write the history of the Bond Club for this site.

Perhaps the most stress relates to my daughter's pending wedding, slated for November 13, 2004. The invitation list has created the most controversy, but usually I am assigned some lesser function such as typing up the directions to the wedding and the reception. These important jobs create just one more pile of havoc. Every time I try to help out with a list, I am chastised for having the wrong zip codes, or incorrect middle initials, or whatever. Nobody can read my handwriting! (For more details, see the chapter on wedding preparations.)

The family dog, Gizmo, is blind and seems to blend in with this maze of materials. At the age of twelve, he has daily drops for his eyes plus a series of other meds. A collection of these items also decorates the card tables. Remnants of card games played with the boys from the Chatham Men's Club constantly need to be organized.

I am somewhat amazed at the flow of "finished product" that actually does emanate from my office. So many late afternoons and early evenings are consumed by off periods that I am forced to take advantage of my on times as best I can. Also, physical therapy or a golf game can be very tiring and time consuming as well.

In short, I maintain a fairly unkempt office. My wife tries to add "pretty things" such as a box of cookies or chocolates, cashews, Sunmaid raisins, paper weights, flashlights, and usually a copy of the newspaper containing some story which fascinates her. Additionally, there is usually one "unauthorized" saltshaker. Sometimes, evidences of my Parkinson's factor are conspicuous as well. My hefti-bag of pills is always near the center of my whole operation. Liquids relating to consuming the pills are woven into this entire fabric. Buried in the mix are my portable phone and the remote for the nearby TV. In fact, one of the difficult items to find is the phone. It is particularly irksome to have the phone ring and be unable to find it. Usually, it lies under some innocuous piece of stationary or simply just blends in with all the piles. Perhaps I should order one in Hertz yellow!

In my mind, everything has its place, and I am content with how my area is set up. As a sole proprietorship, I like the smooth-functioning PAL Publishing Company. The key to the company's relatively modest success is the quality of its end product. To a degree, PAL Publishing thrives on clutter. I also remember the expression from when I worked on Wall Street: "An uncluttered desk is the sign of an uncluttered mind."

Also, my other material is within reach should I have to shift gears from say the BCNJ to LC. Some mornings, the phone is humming from a variety of different sources. Other days are extremely quiet.

My wife likes a very structured living room and dining room area. I feel that she wants to look ready to receive company from any source. She is not too fond of the array of notebooks that sit under my desk. From my standpoint, the different colors and large labels help me classify the notebooks by category so just by knowing its color, I can reach for the right notebook. This is especially meaningful when trying to time a new issue equity trade. In my heart, I know my wife would prefer me to use all one color notebook or use smaller notebooks with each notebook representing a separate category.

My wife is also not too pleased with the computer hardware that supports my writing effort. Items such as modems, power bars, zip drives, and the hard drive of my Dell computer all are connected to my computer screen, keyboard and mouse, and my Hewlett Packard T-45, which is a combination printer, copier, fax machine, and scanner all rolled into one unit. She frequently asks me, "Why are there so many freakin' wires under your desk?"

The number of the various notebooks varies from time to time, but usually I have around ten. I am not pleased with the location of the notebooks (i.e., below my computer desk), as sometimes they're difficult to reach and I strain my back in the process. I wish I had a better system!

Were it not for my Parkinson's ailment, I am sure my wife would insist on a much neater tone to my office. She is obviously aware that I need a ton of material to handle all my various assignments. Actually, when we are expecting company she diplomatically requests that I tidy up my area, and so every once in a while I quickly file all my stuff in assorted boxes or on various clipboards. Once cleaned off, the two card tables become natural locations for any hors d'oeuvres that she might want to serve. It seems we always entertain company in the first of our two living rooms. Somehow, I think outsiders feel more comfortable in a little bit of clutter. At least I do!

Wednesdays are officially declared cleanup day at 8 Carmine Street in Chatham, New Jersey. My wife takes to the war path—every light bulb must be changed, every battery must be checked, and all recycling must be put in the queue. I try to stay out of the way, and frequently schedule a lunch date. My Parkinson's doesn't respond well to pressure, and so I am apt to freeze up more frequently on cleanup day than other more tranquil days. And so, my plans of helping her are foiled by the PD and I lose a lot of potentially useful time while she complains of no sleep and having to do everything. She rattles off a memorized list so fast that I can only write down half of the items.

An example of her neatness syndrome is her treatment of the various photograph albums accumulated over our forty years of marriage. She likes to keep the albums in the second living room, enclosed in cabinets, and strictly arranged in chronological order. She becomes quite upset whenever anyone disturbs the domestic tranquility of this line-up. If the albums are checked out by some of our daughters' friends (the albums are quite entertaining to scan every now and then!), and if they are not precisely returned later on, my wife goes ballistic, yells at me (of course I may indeed be the culprit), and proceeds to take out all the albums and reestablish their proper sequence. In the process, each album and shelf gets a new dusting.

Another fetish, which may not be an extreme, involves her ironing of my most casual of casual shirts and shorts. In Cinnie's book, even tank tops, which I may only wear as underwear, must be ironed. So she stays up late at night, ironing away, and then the next day reports how tired she is.

Filing cabinets and tray organizers seem to work for both of us. I recently bought a tri-level organizer, which sits on my main computer desk. The slick device is neatly arranged to hold the top priority items on my agenda. For example, as I write this chapter, one of the trays holds all the paperwork connected with the Class of 1960 Golf Tourney. A brilliant red envelope contains participants' responses, directions to the golf club, starting times, and their sixty-dollar entrance fees. Another tray houses the wedding invitation list. Once an event takes place, the tray is cleared and another entry is made.

My Hewlet Packard T-45, or Office Jet, also is crucial to my organizational capability. As mentioned above, the unit contains a copier, a scanner, a fax machine, and a printer. As far as I know, the machine retails for around $300 and is worth every penny. Naturally, the computer itself, where a multitude of information is on file via disc, eliminates a huge amount of clutter. I also try to miniaturize whenever I can.

But Parkinson's is the number one, real culprit in this story. At least four times a day, my body is completely rigid and I am unable to do any filing or anything! When I try to file a document while in the off position, my hand just stiffens on the file—I can't move—and I am unable to let the document go into the filing cabinet or even an appropriately neat place. Everywhere I turn I see miniature piles. If I try to disturb them when I am off, there's a distinct possibility I'll knock the entire pile over!

A second cause of clutter in our house is the publications industry. I used to subscribe to many magazines and three newspapers (the *NY Times*, the *Star Ledger*, and the *Chatham Courier*), but recycling requirements have made constant cleanup necessary. On Sundays, the *New York Times* is particularly thick and virtually impossible to read in its entirety before the next morning's paper hits the front lawn. As a result, we cancelled our home delivery of the Sunday edition of the *New York Times* as well as several magazines. As a broad-based common stock investor, I receive annual reports from about thirty to forty companies. For some reason, I receive two editions each week of *Sports Illustrated*.

And then there is that part of me that never wants to throw anything away! For years, I saved the game program from every sports event I attended. Some of these programs have proved very valuable for me now that I am an author (I use the term loosely). For example, such records gave me some somewhat original information from the college basketball era of the 1950s and 1960s, which greatly contributed to my biography of Butch van Breda Kolff.

I noticed that once I was stricken with Parkinson's I gradually began to lose interest in my program collection. This was partly because I kept the collection in the attic. I attempted to preserve the collection with plastic wrap and organized the stacks as best I could in chronological order. But as I grew older, my balance grew suspect. I disliked venturing to the attic just to maintain the file. I had other collections (i.e., baseball caps and long-playing or 33 r.p.m. record albums), but I let them taper off as well. I even began to keep my tax materials downstairs. The aversion

to the attic added to the accumulation of paper in the main living areas. To a lesser extent, my dislike of the stairs leading to the basement also contributed to this pattern.

The Great Society and its emphasis on holidays and birthdays also adds to the inventory of clutter in the form of cards, gifts, and the like. I realize the significance of the Christmas season and other holidays to our domestic economy, but I much prefer Labor Day and Groundhog Day to our so called "big" holidays. If you must offer me a gift, may I suggest a gift certificate for my favorite local restaurant. In the first place, my wife and I enjoy eating out and the certificates are actually more useful than some of the other gifts I receive. Also, I keep a file of the pending certificates in the "magic drawer" of my desk. Gifts that are in the wrong size seem to sit around forever, and some get filed in a drawer somewhere without being returned.

My Bedroom

When one of my daughters graduated college and took a job in Boston, she afforded us the opportunity to "spread out" and possibly attain a better night's sleep. In tandem with my Parkinson's disease, I arise each morning at six a.m. and try to get to bed at ten p.m. On average, I am in bed for seven to eight hours each night.

On the other hand, my wife is more apt to get to bed about one a.m. and arise about nine a.m. I am more of a morning person and she is nocturnal. When Priscilla vacated her double bed, I adopted it as my own. If I have trouble rising from the bed, I have a siren-type alarm that I can use to arouse my wife.

On cleanup day, I am expected to make an extra effort to tidy the house. A lounging chair, which contains a ton of clothes and other personal items, must be arranged to look better. I snag about ten hangers from various closets and then hang up all my shirts.

But cleanup day as it applies to the bedroom disrupts my routine and may cause me some dismay the next morning. For example, to accommodate her vacuuming efforts, Cinnie places all my shoes on the "organizer chair." She also collapses the stationary walker and places it some distance from the bed. If I don't notice these changes before retiring at night, it's possible that I may have difficulty locating my clothing that I intended to wear the next morning.

My wife's thorough management style in all these matters can be a source of stress around the house. She is quite insistent on what she wants and when she wants it achieved. At or near the top of her daily list is the mandatory dispensing of birdseed to our array of feeders in the back yard. Among our aviary visitors, only the male cardinal qualifies as a creature of beauty. Otherwise, an endless collection of New Jersey gray squirrels, wrens, and clones of the Atlantic City pigeon clog the feeding lines in our backyard. What angers me about the chore is that we are supporting the lifestyle of some aggressive squirrels who have found a comfortable nesting locale inside the engine of my Lincoln Continental.

Very recently, while my wife was rushing to get to her job at the Paper Mill Playhouse, she kept urging me to lay out some birdseed in the backyard, When I told her that I was having a Parkinson's freeze-up, she said, "Do it when you are feeling better." I told her that would be fifteen minutes or so, and she said, "OK." But hardly five minutes had passed, and she asked me when was I going to feed the birds. She obviously recognized my irritation with the animals that were wrecking my car!

I told her that I was still frozen and that it would be probably another ten or fifteen minutes. Finally, following yet another request, I lost my patience and grabbed the birdseed as best I could. On my first trip, I almost fell on the frozen tundra left by a recent snow-storm. At last I was "defrosted," when my pills became effective, and I tried again. I was then able to scatter the seed evenly along the path to the feeders.

Fortunately, I have a lot of other items on my daily agenda. Otherwise, retirement with Parkinson's would be for the birds.

As I write about the house in Chatham, my mind drifts back to when we moved to Chatham some thirty-seven years ago. The talk of the town was the Newcomers Club, and so my wife and I joined. We instantly were thrust into an active social life of others in their thirties, most of whom had young children (though we did not), and fairly decent jobs on Wall Street or with nearby ATT. The group held a regular schedule of rotational dinners, whereby you went to one member's house for cocktail hour, another member hosted dinner, and a third provided the venue for desert and after-dinner drinks. One of our first friends in this organization was Larry O'-Hearn and his wife June. In fact, June was president of the Newcomers Club when we first joined.

On August 14, 2004, Larry O'Hearn died at the age of seventy-two following a twenty-year battle with Parkinson's disease. His obituary listed his many activities and positions, truly recognizing his role as an active Parkinsonian.

He was a member of the Naval Reserves for twenty years and was the past commodore of the Normandy Beach Yacht Club. He was a past trustee of the Library of the Chathams. He was president of the Chatham Board of Health and a trustee of the Minisink Swim Club. When I knew him best, he was with Smith Barney, but he subsequently retired from Wheat First Securities, where he was a senior vice president. He specialized in institutional equities.

I admired Larry's activities, but I also enjoyed some of the personal comments listed in the obituary. His family noted that Larry was "a true gentleman in every way, and always had a kind word for everyone." The article also said he was a mentor to young people and a "proud father." Ironically, Larry's obituary listed the Parkinson Foundation as an outlet for memorial contributions. The address given was 710 West 168th St. in New York, the exact building where I participated in the Columbia University research project and where I was a patient of Dr. Cheryl Waters.

Another active Parkinsonian in our lives was Louise Conklin, who died in 2005 at the age of sixty-seven. Her obituary read that she had a long struggle with Lewy Body Dementia, a condition long associated with PD. Louise was president of the League of Women Voters of Chatham, and while she was in office, my wife was in charge of the organization's finance drive.

Chapter 7A

Vacation I

The use of the word "vacation" is a little misleading, because I am supposedly retired from the business world. Theoretically, my life should be a *permanent* vacation, and traveling should ebb and flow as a natural consequence of the overall retirement process. But somehow, the demands of my little publishing company plus my wife's active role at the Paper Mill Playhouse and related telemarketing firms created the need to simply get away. Yet another cold, inclement winter in the Northeast made the need to escape to a warmer climate even more compelling. In many respects, we needed to get away from our daily routines just to maintain our sanity.

In our younger years, when considering the location of our next vacation, we ambitiously focused on islands in the Caribbean. We rarely revisited these island paradises, and tended to try something new on each vacation junket. Sometimes even an excursion to Mexico worked into our plans. On the Caribbean Island circuit, over the years we stayed in Anguila, Antigua,

Aruba, Bahamas, Barbados, British West Indies, Cayman Islands, Jamaica, Nevis, Puerto Rico, St. Kitts, St. Maartan's, U.S. Virgin Islands (i.e., St. Croix, St. John's, and St. Thomas), and perhaps the tiniest of them all, St. Barts. To get to St. Barts, we connected on a small four-passenger plane. My wife and I were the only two on board other than the pilot, and it felt as if we were floating like a kite on a string. We held hands all the way from the airport in Charlotte Amelia (St. Thomas) to the tiny airstrip in St. Barts.

Our Mexican adventures included Cancun, Mexico City, Acapulco, and Puerto Vejarta.

Planning Ahead

But now, with my Parkinson's condition, such traveling requires immensely more planning. Unlike the pre-PD days, I couldn't just throw a few items into the suitcase and be ready to roll in a matter of an hour or two. For one vacation, because I had put on a lot of weight, I had to try on clothes for several days to make sure what I was packing actually fit me. Clothing featuring elastic waists were most in demand. Then folding and packing the items squarely in the suitcase became a problem. No matter how I tried, I couldn't seem to flatten and fold my clothes along any sort of crease. So, the Sunday before we were to fly, Raymond helped me pack all the items I wanted to bring. He accomplished this basically easy function in a matter of minutes, and I was set to roll. My wife kept finding more suitable clothes, but I didn't want to mess with Raymond's packing scheme. All my shorts and tank tops fit nicely into two modestly-sized bags. I had packed enough clothing for three times the length of our stay anyway!

My plan was to leave the bags at the curbside check-in at the airport, and I would use a ditty bag to carry on my meds and any other last minute items.

I had fresh supplies of all my Parkinson's pills. I pre-counted the pills to make sure the number of pills I was bringing more than covered the 250 pills I would take over the next eleven days.

Anticipating a possible interview with the *Newark Star Ledger* business section upon my return from Florida, I brought a copy of my book about the Howard Savings Bank entitled, *Howard Powerless.* Because I started writing books almost three years earlier, I needed to refresh myself on some of its contents. My Parkinson's memory could be amazing in the recall of detail. It also could draw a big blank!

Because of my Parkinson's factor, in recent years we have limited experimental traveling and elected to return to places that we liked and that accommodated our curtailed lifestyle. Our three favorite resorts include: Key Biscayne Florida (The Sonesta Beach Hotel), Key West Florida (The Pier House), and Fort Lauderdale (Florida Largo Mer).

My condition necessitates that we stay at a full service resort. When just the two of us are traveling, we need help with our luggage when we check into and out of our resort. I carry a separate billfold of five-dollar and one-dollar bills strictly to tip porters, bellmen, and airport agents. Having the gratuity money at hand is a lot better than fumbling around for my wallet only to

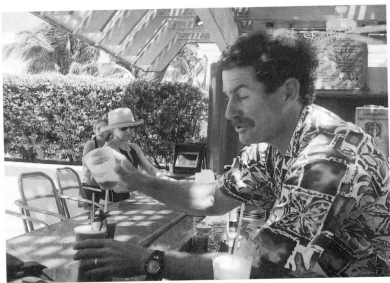

Gino is the manager of the Sonesta Hotel's renowned Pool Bar. His rum drinks are famous as he siphons the run through the upper reaches of the appropriate straw.

find all I have are twenty-dollar bills available. Before tipping too generously, I find out if a gratuity fee is added onto the bill at the resort.

All three resorts listed above have activities that are readily at hand. Breakfast, lunch, and dinner—and even room service—are available every day. We have an innate distaste for deadlines in the dining and shopping areas.

For our 2004 vacation, we selected Key Biscayne, which is a fairly developed island connected by the Rickenbacker Causeway to the city of Miami. In the 1960s, KB sprang into the limelight when Richard Nixon used his home there as the summer White House retreat for his presidency. Key Biscayne is also the location of the Seaquarium, home of the moviestar dolphin Flipper. The golf and tennis facilities on the island are excellent and have been the scene of several professional tournaments.

In 1994, Key Biscayne faced near destruction in the wake of Hurricane Andrew. During this massively destructive storm, the Hotel Sonesta stood like a fortress while others nearby were totally ruined. It took the island about four to five years to recover from Andrew.

The Day Before the flight

My wife was indeed in a "tizzy" the day before the flight. The all-important appointment with the hair dresser loomed in the middle of the day, our cleaning person had decided to come this day instead of the day before, Cinnie had scheduled two sessions of ushering at the Paper Mill Playhouse, and she was trying to buy our younger daughter Priscilla some presents for her birthday, which would take place the day after we returned. Then, the carpenter in charge of our kitchen renovation, a more-or-less ongoing project, paid us a surprise visit with all sorts of new suggestions. Cinnie also prepared three meals for me.

At about ten p.m., my luggage was neatly stacked by the front door, where it would rest for the evening. I was quite relaxed about having everything in order for the flight. Phil, our dependable family limo driver, would pick us up at ten-thirty a.m. the next day.

I believe it was between two a.m. and three a.m. when I heard my wife's footsteps traversing the hard wooden floors of our attic overhead, no doubt looking for her suitcase to pack for Florida. Her suitcase was huge and impossible to carry down the attic staircase. So she slid it down the steps, creating a loud thumping noise that pierced the serenity of the early morning air. Beyond that episode, though, she was packed in a flash and her suitcase was soon positioned properly in the middle of the living room. Although she would catch little sleep, she was ready to roll. She slept until almost nine-thirty a.m.

As anticipated, Phil was punctual in the discharge of his limo duties. Since being ruled a non-driver, I have used Phil more and more to simply get me places. We have always enjoyed his pleasant company, and he is welcome to come into our house and retrieve all our luggage. Other drivers always seemed to expect us to at least carry the bags to the front stoop or the curb!

Phil's car was a 1995 Lincoln Town Car that showed 142,000 miles on the odometer. My wife truly liked the comfort of the mint-condition vehicle, and considered buying it as a replacement for her own 1991 Chevrolet Caprice station wagon with some 250,000 miles logged thereon. But for some reason, when Phil mentioned he was thinking of selling the car and replacing it with a new one—as a means of updating the image of his company—she mentioned that she too would opt for a new car when her busy schedule permitted.

At any rate, we arrived at the American Airlines terminal at Newark Airport about eleven a.m., and we immediately requested a wheelchair from the porter who was about to check our luggage. At the same time, I also requested a wheelchair to meet me when we arrived in Miami. Soon, the porter had us en route to our gate with an agent who pushed me along in the wheelchair. We discharged Phil for the day, and reconfirmed that we would see him upon our return. I was amazed at how little traffic there was at the outdoor check-in facility.

The next step was the security checkpoint, which essentially was a scene of organized chaos. Though I was obviously handicapped—I really couldn't do much in the way of hijacking—the security staff was very thorough in investigating my body and travel bag for any weapons or metal devices. I removed my shoes and walking brace when I was unable to pass through the electronic gate without sounding the alarm. After a modest delay, my metallic belt buckle was ruled the culprit. I was truly glad I was on during this entire experience, or we might have missed our flight. At long last, we collected all of our carry-on material and were on our way to Gate 33 where our plane would soon take off for Florida. Since wheelchairs cannot negotiate escalators, we had to take a series of elevators to arrive at our destination.

In the pre-planning of our trip, we had requested an aisle seat as close to the front of the plane as possible. American Airlines accommodated me with seat 7H, which was just behind the first class section and next to the lavatory. Also, the American agent gave the handicapped passengers early boarding privileges, which helped us get organized before the rest of the some 250 passengers sought their seats.

For the two or three weeks prior to the Key Biscayne trip, I had harbored all kinds of thoughts about what could go wrong. Once I was belted into seat 7H, I finally let myself relax. I felt great, actually, and so I ordered a chardonnay to celebrate the start of our vacation. I even used one of the five-dollar bills that I had stashed in my left-hand sports jacket pocket. Somewhere en route, midway through my cocktail, I must have dozed off. The three-hour flight went by quickly, and soon the captain was telling us over the loudspeaker to prepare for landing. I suddenly realized that my condition had changed from being on to being off. When I get relaxed or am otherwise preoccupied, I tend to lose focus and forget my pills. Before I could take my catch-up potion, there I was, with a potential audience of more than 250 passengers, frozen solid.

Gradually, as the effects of the chardonnay wore off and the pills started to pull me back to on, I became less rigid. I had to wait for the entire passenger load to deplane before I could seek my wheelchair connection to the baggage claim area. The experience was somewhat socially embarrassing but soon corrected.

Miami International Airport has to be one of the world's largest and busiest! It seemed it would take an eternity to work our way from the plane to the baggage area. Despite its size, there seem to be a shortage of elevators. Therefore, all the handicapped passengers from all the flights were forced to squeeze through the United States Customs Department, site of the only convenient elevator. Because we were domestic passengers passing through customs, we were not allowed to be accompanied by our spouses or traveling aides. In a hurried transaction, I handed my wife her flight ticket and passport ID and said I would meet her at the train to the baggage department in a few minutes. She was headed for the escalator, I was headed for the elevator. Theoretically, our separate ventures would reunite us at the entrance to the short railroad ride to the baggage claim area.

When the airport agent and I opened the elevator door, we were greeted by a sea of humanity swirling in every direction. We looked for my wife where we thought she should have landed, but she wasn't there. Suddenly, a uniformed guard came over to me and mentioned that there was this hysterical woman who had lost her husband. There was my wife, some thirty yards from us, shielded from us by this massive flow of people. Soon we were rejoined, and we were off for the train to the baggage claim area. Only one more crisis occurred. When my wife asked me the whereabouts of our plane tickets and passports, I said that I had handed them to her shortly after the elevator-escalator episode. For a minute she panicked, and then started to cry as she envisioned the impossible mission of retracing our steps to the plane. Fortunately, she found the envelope within her shopping bag/carry-on filing system.

Finally, we were at the baggage claim where, as pre-arranged, the ubiquitous Raymond and his pal Kelly were there to greet us. The twosome would be staying at a small hotel on Key Biscayne for about six days. Given our delays arising from my freeze-up and my lost wife, Kelly had already taken our luggage off the turnstile. After yet another modest delay caused by the heavy volume of airport auto traffic, we were headed for our final destination, the Sonesta Beach Hotel. Soon, we were checked into our corner room, Room 448.

Room 448 at the Sonesta Beach Hotel

The Sonesta is an imposing structure and dwarfs the other buildings in the immediate area. Its quasi-pyramid appearance enables the hotel to provide many balcony rooms facing directly toward Biscayne Bay. Room 448 was just such a room and featured a wrap-around balcony. Although we requested a handicapped room, we thought we could adapt to our environment because of the balcony.

On most of our past travels, we had become accustomed to changing rooms at least once during a stay at any given resort. But since we had stayed in an equivalent room only a year or so prior, we were unlikely to change rooms on this trip.

The room was located about as far from the elevator as you could get. It seemed as if I had to walk at least the length of one football field before reaching our room. I paced off seventy-six steps between the entrance to the elevator and our doorway. The officially classified handicapped rooms, which were available but lacked balconies, were located directly at the elevator corridor. I rationalized that the extra walk would help get me in shape and perhaps work off some of the surplus weight I was carrying.

After giving the room a cursory inspection, the four of us proceeded to the dining room for an early dinner. There was no luncheon on the flight down, although my wife had made us each a sandwich to tide us over. We ate dinner in the cocktail lounge called Desires. While ordering off the bar menu, we could also watch the NBA play-offs on TV. This option was especially important to sports fanatic Raymond. Following dinner, we returned to Room 448. We were stalled in our efforts to open the door when our plastic key produced nothing but red and amber lights in the door-lock mechanism.

To no avail, we all tried various keys and angles. Fortunately, the night maid spotted our frustration, and she let us into the room with her pass key. She informed the front desk of our problem and they stamped out another set of keys, which were forwarded up to my wife and me.

The next morning offered us another perfect day in Paradise, without a cloud in the sky and eighty-degree weather. We decided to take it easy and sit by the pool after such a hectic travel day. But we needed some items from the room, so after breakfast we returned to Room 448. Again, we inserted the new plastic keys and they, like their predecessors, were ineffective in charging the green light needed to open the door. Like déjà vu, the maid who was about to make up our room let us in. This time, we decided to call the front desk and register a complaint about the door mechanism.

The solution was very basic. The door mechanism needed new batteries. We were surprised that routine maintenance checks hadn't detected the problem, but we weren't going to let this minor inconvenience get to us.

The Chest of Drawers

The bathroom in Room 448 was reasonably large and contained a closet with a small wall safe that we used to stow our valuables. The odd piece of furniture in the bathroom was this rather large chest of drawers. The chest featured six drawers, which tapered down in size from top to bottom. As a piece of furniture, it was quite simple in style, hardly befitting an expensive hotel like the Sonesta. It resembled a piece you might find in a college dormitory, and appeared as if it had been constructed from a kit. The standard issue coffee pot sat on top of the piece. I claimed the bureau for my clothes, as this would be an easy way for me to get ready early in the morning without waking my wife in the other room. But as I stocked the chest of drawers, I noticed that the piece had a tendency to be a bit wobbly. I wondered if the workman who constructed the bureau had tightened all the screws! When I put some clothes in the top drawer, the entire unit leaned forward. Regardless, I wanted to get off to the beach, and so I packed the bureau with all the clothes I had brought.

The first time I wanted to change clothes, I invaded the drawers and took out some underwear for underneath my bathing suit. As I attempted to balance myself and put my left foot into my underwear, I leaned on the edge of the bureau. Immediately, the bureau started to crash down on me and I had to hold up the fully-loaded piece or face serious injury should it collapse on top of me. Simultaneously, the coffee pot crashed to the floor and shattered on the bathroom tile. I screamed for help, and Raymond (who was on the phone in the next room) came to my rescue. Together, we righted the bureau. Once we had the area squared away, Raymond—an experienced rectifier—was on the phone with the front desk informing them of the near horror show. He demanded a new bureau for Room 448.

A team of maintenance men quickly came up to the room, and instead of replacing the bureau, welded the back into the wall and solidified its position. The newly secured bureau withstood the pressure tests applied by the heavier members of the maintenance team. Meanwhile, as I sat trembling in my chair, I thanked God that Raymond was nearby at the time of the incident. For real, I don't know how long I could have held that bureau on my own!

The Bed in Room 448

For the first night, when we both were pretty exhausted from all the events that had taken place, my wife and I slept fairly soundly, oblivious to any problems involving the bed. The structure was king-sized and involved a strongly constructed headboard. The second night, however, as I prepared to go to bed for the night, I noticed the maid had manufactured a championship series of hospital corners and had turned down the bedding so as to have them on prominent display. My preference in the realm of sheets is for a loose tuck so that I can readily turn over in the night. My limited mobility comes to a halt at night, and maneuvering a tightly locked hospital corner is not a joy for me. And so I untidied the bed and my wife told the maid to skip the hospital corners for the balance of the stay. To a large extent, the bed was cooperative and didn't disrupt our sleep. I had some difficulty getting out of bed, but my wife gave me a hand and I was on my way.

After a few runs to the bathroom, we had a routine that enabled us to sleep in relative comfort free of worry about during-the-night accidents.

As our vacation progressed, we got to know the people at the front desk on a first name basis, because of the following events.

- We had a mini-bar refrigerator conk out and need to be replaced. Because we were using the unit to store some perishable goods to make my wife's hors d'oeuvres, the hotel gave us an entirely separate refrigerator for our own use independent of the mini-bar operation. There was no extra charge for the fridge.

- We had the toilet overflow in the middle of the night, and we had to arouse housekeeping to get some extra towels to clean up the bathroom.
- We had several conversations about the air-conditioning system that keyed into the porch door. All doors and windows had to be locked for the AC to come on. Frequently, it felt like the AC was on, but was only recycling the cooler night air through its vents. We preferred to sleep with the doors open and the AC off, but this recycling effect made it seem like the AC was blasting cold air on us. This problem self-corrected when the outdoor air warmed up later on during our trip.
- The AC formed a condensation that dripped all night and left a moist area between the bedroom and the bathroom.

After a few days, we had most all the problems with the room under control. The hotel was gracious in its sympathy for our inconvenience and gave us one night free during our stay. The weather was near perfect (only one rainout day) and we quickly exhibited our newly-acquired Florida tans.

Dining

One night, early in the trip, we ate diner exceptionally late and my freeze-up set in about ten p.m. When it came time to sign the check, I was totally in a locked position. Raymond had to work my walker backward through the crowd so I could exit the restaurant. After that, in deference to my PD, we were more punctual and generally speaking ate dinner in the seven-thirty to eight o'clock range. We had a little difficulty at the extremely popular Rusty Pelican restaurant. The food and the service were great, but it took forever on a Saturday night to extricate our rental car from the valet parking attendants. While waiting on line for our car, the crowd of local diners was very courteous when they saw me freeze up, and they urged me to the head of the line. For the PD victim, a few minutes can make such a difference.

We found one restaurant to be particularly to our liking, and so we returned there three times in our ten days on Key Biscayne. *La Piazzetta* was its name, and the food was delicious. Dinner for four, including gratuities, averaged $150, which seemed in line with resort community pricing. On our last night, when we were anxious to return to our room and get packed, the management of the restaurant was especially kind to us when we were unable to catch a cab for at least thirty minutes. The manager actually offered us a ride home in his personal BMW. I guess that was just reward for our being "customer of the week."

Games

With few exceptions, such as golf, very little in the way of athletic endeavor is possible for the advanced PD victim. Beach volleyball and jogging on the beach are just not that feasible, although swimming might work for some. I found it hard to execute my once somewhat coordinated swimming stroke.

Even the concept of lying in the sun, hour after hour, especially when combined with two or three pina coladas from the bar, no longer had any appeal to me.

I liked being outside, however, and playing a card game by the name of Skip-Bo and a word game called Scattergories was quite an entertaining way to pass the time. The adjustments were made, and we sat under the limited cover of the pool-bar deck, drank virgin pina coladas, and engrossed ourselves in some three-to-four hour sessions of these games.

As for the card game Skip-Bo, I was quite competitive once I learned the rules and as long as my condition was on. The game requires an element of concentration whereby the player must focus on several open stacks of cards as possible discards. You try to reach your discard from the primary deck as soon as possible, and the player who discarded this entire stack (thirty cards or so) first was declared the winner. Blocking techniques, avoiding burying reusable cards, and maximizing use of the Skip-Bo cards (i.e., wild cards) all enter into the strategies of different players.

During this particular vacation, my difficulties came when my off cycle hit. It became very difficult for me to pick up cards from the deck, and to concentrate on my various options. Raymond and Kelly essentially walked me through these rounds, and I even won a couple of games while off.

The game Scattergories is action-oriented and while we were in Key Biscayne my wife frequently joined us as a fourth participant. For each round of play, you see twelve categories such as "amphibious mammals" or "foreign capitals," and within a three-minute span you are expected to list a representative of said category beginning with the letter of choice for the round. A multi-sided cube has most of the letters of the alphabet registered, and the letter of the round is determined by a roll of the cube. If the letter "C" had been rolled, then "crocodile" would be OK for the amphibious mammal while "Cairo" would fit for a foreign capital. It behooves each player to be a little more original in his response for each category, because no points are given for a tie or duplicate selection.

Again, I had no trouble with Scattergories, and even tended to win most of the games. That is, when I was in on mode. As I drifted toward off. I had difficulty writing my answers on the score sheet, especially beyond the fourth answer of the round. Clever answers that popped into my brain when I was on were just not happening. Generally speaking, I averaged eight or more right answers when on, around four (with many no-responses) when I was off.

As the vacation wore on, we became more excited about Skip-Bo than Scattergories. Scattergories was too repetitive, and we kept duplicating answers for the same letters and categories. In my spare time, I pledged to create some new and humorous categories to make the game a little more stimulating.

Skip-Bo, however, evolved into some tenacious battles. We played most of the time as a three-man game, and when one player got way ahead, the other two would work in unison to block his progression toward going out. The cards were sometimes "hot," sometimes "cold," and all three of us were guilty of overlooking some obvious plays available to us.

I also tried to do the crossword puzzles each day in the *Miami Herald* and the *New York Times*. As you may know, these puzzles are challenging to begin with, but get increasingly difficult as the week wears on. I also try to tackle the crossword provided in my airline's magazine. The rest of the group indulged in the jumbo scrabble puzzle provided each day in the *Herald*.

I scheduled one round of golf and then cancelled when I had all kinds of negative thoughts about my ability to keep up with the other three members of an anonymous foursome. My pals who play with me in New Jersey are sympathetic and allow me to hit Mulligans (i.e., do-overs) and to forgo shots from awkward areas of the course (i.e., sand traps, ravines, etc). I also had zero equipment with me on the trip, and I would have had to rent shoes, golf clubs, and a golf cart as well as pay greens fees and buy a ton of balls.

Florida golf courses are known for water, wind, and sand traps. Balls hit into the water are called "gator bait." The course at Key Biscayne featured water on almost every hole. It might have cost me $200 to play one torturous round of golf. I got a haircut instead.

Incidentally, my fears about golf were a bit unfounded. The following Friday I played somewhat competitive golf at a Lafayette College outing and basically held my own in a scramble format. The team used my drive on the par three holes. On the other hand, as you will see in the chapter entitled "What Lies Ahead," I have had some unfortunate experiences on the golf course as well.

The Trip Home

Monday May 4 was a terrible weather day up and down the east coast of the United States, with the possible exception of sunny southern Florida. Our flight from

Miami to Newark was slated for a comfortable two-thirty p.m., and we again opted for the wheelchair at the curbside check-in and used an agent to guide us through the security section. Indeed, the Miami staff was every bit as thorough as their counterparts in Newark. One of the agents in security was a six foot, five inch man who looked like he played tackle for the Miami Dolphins. He approached me, put on a pair of white gloves, and informed me that he was going to frisk me from head to toe. Indeed he did! Once satisfied that I was not a terrorist, he told me to gather my belongings, which I had emptied from my pockets prior to meeting up with him. I just hoped anything of value (wallet, watch, passport, tickets, keys, etc.) was still with us. Given the confusion and activity of the security area, it pays to travel light!

Once we arrived at our gate area, we learned that the flight would be delayed thirty minutes because of weather problems along the route. We would soon board the plane and be en route to Newark, New Jersey, where the weather was rainy, windy, and cold (55 degrees). The flight was bumpy and the flight captain advised us to keep our seat belts on the entire trip. The delay of the flight caused me to be a bit off schedule with my pills, but I was fine when we landed and went for our luggage. My wheelchair agent was a very attractive woman and she stayed with us until Phil could swing the Lincoln around to the pick-up area. Within twenty minutes or so, we were at our front door in Chatham.

Because our mail had been organized and prioritized while we were away, it was easy to get back into bill-paying mode. It didn't take long for the problems we had left behind, the problems we had forgotten about, to resurface and reestablish our irritable moods.

For months, I had been expressing an interest in possibly moving to Florida. The warm weather was the main attraction. At the age of sixty-six, I figured that there would only be a few more good years left before the PD got a lot worse.

Chapter 7B

Vacation II

When we checked into Room 522 at the Lago Mar Resort in Fort Lauderdale (Florida), we were immediately impressed by the size of the suite, the vistas from the balconies on two sides of the room, the monstrous king-sized bed, and the sleek bathroom featuring a black marble—almost glass-like—floor along with a walk-in shower and as many mirrors as you could possibly need. Although functionally designated as a handicapped unit, the tasteful motif of the room seemed to incorporate the overall style of the Lago Mar, which featured a weaving sequence of pools and palm trees as we viewed the properties from the top of the complex. In many respects, Lago Mar was like an isolated yet self-sufficient campus of Floridian luxury and beauty. As previous and frequent visitors to the Lago Mar, we had come to expect it to be a high quality backdrop for our stay in Fort Lauderdale. Regardless, my wife and I were immediately pleased with our new home for the next eight days. This time, our trip would be a lot different.

161

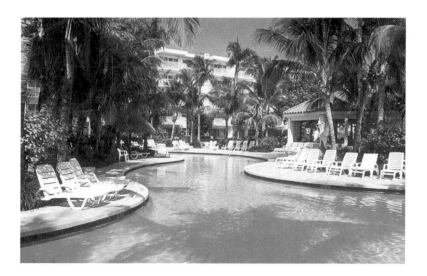

Actually, Room 522 was one of only two handicapped-equipped suites available at the Lago Mar. Unlike at many hotel facilities, Lago Mar handicapped guests had no bathtub to climb over in order to reach the shower line. A very subtle tilt of the shower floor enabled most of the shower water to flow to the drain. A special chair was provided as well as a rinsing device that allowed the handicapped person the possibility of reaching remote portions of his or her body. Pull-up bars were installed on either side of the toilet seat, which was higher than the norm.

To many, Fort Lauderdale is synonymous with the collegiate phenomenon known as spring break. In the 1960s, the popular song by recording star Connie Francis entitled *Where the Boys Are* and its movie counterpart by the same name depicted Fort Lauderdale as a city swarming with bare-chested, somewhat inebriated

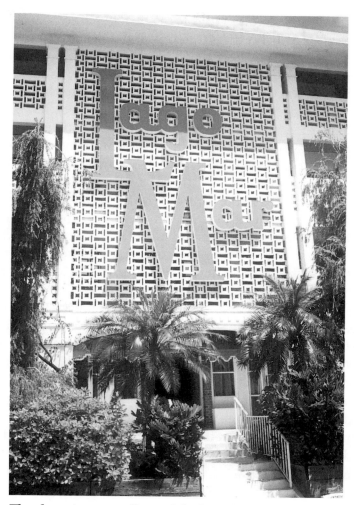

*The elegant surroundings of the Lago Mar Resort in
Fort Lauderdale, Florida were a favorite retreat of the
Luscombe family for several years.
(Photo credit: Paul Luscombe)*

college boys roaming the local beach while searching for young girls on the same mission. Estimates are that the population of Fort Lauderdale peaked somewhere around 1985 when some 350,000 students packed themselves into the local hotels, in some cases boarding twelve students to a room.[1] But the excesses led local leaders to some restrictive reforms. The spring break phenomenon spread to a variety of other resort areas, most notably Miami's South Beach, Key West, and Cancun (Mexico).

At any rate, in the summer of 2004, we had no immediate concerns about bands of spring breakers reveling in the middle of the night. At the Lago Mar Resort, we were more concerned with quieting the sound of the crickets and other night creatures living outside our balcony.

When we turned on the TV to check the local weather, we became somewhat skeptical of the tropical disturbances in the area as we watched the first named storm of 2004—Alex—make a course which would lead to landfall near Cape Hatteras, North Carolina. We more or less assumed the worst had passed the Fort Lauderdale environs, and we decided to change for dinner. Given our modest fatigue from the travel day and the threat of rain outside, we decided to eat in the hotel dining room.

As we prepared to call it a day, a new bed and the need to cross the distance to the toilet required some planning before I retired for the evening. Frankly, I was quite nervous about trying to walk across the slick floor

---

[1]Fodors

without some assistance from my wife. Although at home I would frequently make bathroom trips in the middle of the night without any assistance, I was concerned about the potential for falling on the slick bathroom floor at Lago Mar. Each trip across the floor reminded me of an ice skating rink! I decided I had better use my four-wheeled walker to get me to the critical area in front of the toilet. Towels strewn across the floor seemed to obstruct the movement of the walker.

Before we arrived at the Lago Mar on this trip, we had no idea that the floor would be so slippery. Following an evening of traversing the ice-like surface, my wife called the manager and expressed her concerns about the treacherous situation she felt existed in our room. The manager's office made no suggestions as to how to address the potentially dangerous floor situation in Room 522.

The next morning, anxious to get going on my physical training program, I was an early bird at the Lago Mar Spa. My friend Raymond Monroe joined me and we rode the exercise bike for ten minutes and I did the treadmill for five minutes. I tried some work with a five-pound weight, but that didn't feel so great! Raymond and I then headed for breakfast, a daily feast indeed.

Our first full day was relatively sun-filled, and we tried to grab as many rays as possible. Raymond and I played a ton of cards throughout the day while my wife started her routine of writing all our friends postcards. The next day, Kelly Dodson joined us, bringing an array of other games for us to play poolside. Additionally, we all competitively worked on the newspaper's word games. It seemed that Raymond tried to get the entire Lago Mar staff involved and to checking out some "marginal" words, he daily borrowed the Webster's dictionary from the telephone operator.

Ping-pong, tennis, and miniature golf rounded out the game competition. Kelly and Raymond were about even in ping-pong, while Kelly's superior conditioning led him to an advantage on the tennis court. As expected, I challenged them both at golf, but Raymond's miracle shot on the final green from the bushes into the hole stole the show!

On our second day, we were cruising along in the sun until a dark cloud passed overhead and dumped a heavy volume of water on us. We dashed for the nearby pool bar, and set up our game table under the roof of the open-air structure. Somehow, it seemed that almost everyone staying at the Lago Mar was packed into the bar area. We chatted at length with some lady golfers from Alabama, one of whom chanted the Auburn University fight cheer, which rings out "WAR EAGLE."

The newfound fellowship led to my willingness to have a few cocktails while waiting for the storm to pass, effectively compromising the no-drinking policy that I had enacted to maximize the effectiveness of my PD medicines. But as this weather pattern was repeated over the next few days, I indulged in the likes of pina coladas, orangecycles, banchies, margaritas, banana daiquiris, and chardonnay. I sensed a minimal impact on my behavior, but nothing disastrous happened. For example, I found myself rigidifying closer to nine p.m. rather than ten p.m., and so I headed to bed early on several occasions.

With further rain in the forecast, Cinnie and Kelly set out for the stores to do some food shopping. Later in the week, Cinnie got her hair done at the Galleria Mall near Saks Fifth Avenue, and then we all went with her to Banana Republic, Gap, and Dillard's department store for some vacation-wear purchases. I made my contribution to the local economy with some purchases at the Men's Shop at Lago Mar. Reflecting my continuously bulging waistline, I purchased a pair of size 42 Bermuda shorts. It marked the first time in my life that I wore a 42 waist.

Dinner at the Riverside Hotel

Los Olos Boulevard is the showcase for Fort Lauderdale's most elegant shopping and eating establishments, somewhat resembling Palm Beach's Worth Avenue or Beverly Hills' Rodeo Drive. Los Olos is the setting for the Riverside Hotel; the Grill Room Restaurant located inside the hotel is regarded as one of the city's finest. In celebration of my sixty-sixth birthday, we decided to have dinner there on Tuesday night, August 2 (my birthday really is July 30).

Tuesday evenings are not that busy, and when I told the maitre d'hotel that we would like a table for four, he inquired if we minded sitting near the piano player. Quite the contrary, we seized the opportunity, and once seated, we were within a few feet of the marvelous sounds emanating from the piano. The piano player was a tall, dark-complected Argentine, probably about forty years old, whose long black hair was tied in a pony-tail. He seemed totally consumed by his music, physically pouring himself into the piano. He indeed played with a passion.

The menu was quite pricey, but we were oblivious to the cost of the evening. We were there and why ruin the whole night! The meter was always running, however, as everything was *a la carte*. Cinnie and Raymond ordered filet mignon, while I ordered the snapper. Kelly ordered roast beef, which was unfortunately grilled and not baked. We all avoided appetizers to somewhat contain the final tab.

Vegetables family style plus combinations of potatoes filled out our main courses.

Throughout the evening, up to the completion of our main course, Raymond was very busy away from the table. I figured he was smoking more than his normal amount, but I was soon to enjoy the fruits of his efforts. As the lights dimmed, the piano player started to play the familiar verses of *Happy Birthday,* and soon the head waiter was carrying a beautiful chocolate cake with multicolored blossoms on top. Three candles decorated the top of the cake, and I blew them out happily. Upon completion of the cake ceremony, Raymond and Kelly handed me shopping bags full of presents. I was indeed surprised and sincerely touched by the generosity of my young friends. We each had a slice of cake and, upon returning to the Lago Mar, donated the balance to the staff of the hotel.

The next night we elected to dine at Shula's Steak Restaurant. The legendary Dolphin football coach was not on the scene that evening. A multitude of television sets featuring sports events lined the walls. Cinnie was quite upset with the TV earmarked for our area. In effect, the huge screen was divided into four quadrants delineated with lines across and up and down the screen. She registered a complaint, but the waitress informed us that the lines were a permanent part of the design of the TV set.

The tension between the waitress and Cinnie magnified when my wife discovered that almost all the food at Shula's was filled with garlic, pepper, or some other spice. Although the waitress assured Cinnie that almost any dish could be prepared without garlic, potentially with any sauce placed on the side, Cinnie kept repeating that she's allergic to garlic. Raymond likewise has all kinds of allergies and he too seemed to wear on the waitress with his specifications. Soon, the food order was in and we all enjoyed the meal, once it was prepared and delivered to each one's liking.

The Rustic Crab was the earthiest restaurant on our list. Located just south of the Fort Lauderdale airport, it featured old newspapers as the tablecloths and hammered mallets to signal your waitress or celebrate someone's birthday. Cinnie ordered a Maine lobster, and landlubbers Raymond and Kelly were indeed intrigued by the technique used to dissect the beast. Raymond assisted Cinnie by using the mallets to crush portions of the lobster shell, enabling her to scoop out the sweet lobster meat. Playing defensive Parkinson's strategy, I chose the least difficult item to carve—crab cakes—as my main course.

After dinner, Raymond was totally infatuated with the celebrity photos on the wall at the popular restaurant. Pictures of Marilyn Monroe (nee Norma Jean Baker) particularly caught his eye. We also enjoyed chatting with the manager of the restaurant, who went on frequent hunting trips for thirteen-foot long alligators in the Everglades.

The Incident at the Soda Shop

On one of the rainy mornings, Raymond and I were circulating on the Lago Mar properties when I suggested that we stop at the soda shop to see if they had any football magazines or perhaps some games for us to play while passing time during the bad weather. Raymond bought and wrote some postcards while I bought and skimmed through the abbreviated local version of the *New York Times*. Upon spotting the soda case, I remembered that Cinnie wanted some Diet Sprite, but that the soda shop had been all out when she had checked earlier in the week. But on this morning, I spotted what appeared to be a six-pack of her preferred soda way in back of the soda case on the lowest level, tucked into the rear behind other beverages. When Raymond finished writing the cards to his sisters, I asked him to see if he could reach the Diet Sprite cans in the remote section of the soda case. He indicated he would give it a try in a few minutes, as soon as he checked out some of the inventory available in the gift shop.

In just a few short minutes, I heard a crashing sound and then Raymond's penetrating voice yelling, "Help me! Help me!" When I looked over at the soda case, there was Raymond sitting on the floor with his right arm virtually crushed by a collapsed wall of milk bottles and canned sodas from about three full shelves. One of the attendants from the soda shop quickly moved over to Raymond's side, and one-by-one removed the sodas and bottles from his arm.

We all stood in shock, fearing the worst—that Raymond had broken his arm.

Raymond, though, remained calmer than the several ladies who worked at the soda shop. They were stunned, but one succeeded in calling the front desk. The manager on duty was quickly in the soda shop and he asked Raymond if he needed medical attention. For the time being, Raymond decided to tough it out. He was inwardly angry at whoever stacked the sodas and bottles without securing the platform holding the second level of bottles and cans. He even thought that the tray might have been jerry-rigged just to create the incident.

Earlier in the week, I had called one of my old Lafayette classmates—Joel Gustafson—in hopes of gathering some information for my next class correspondent column in the *Alumni News.* In prior years when I had called his office, Joel was always very busy with his legal practice. But this time, as a recent retiree, he had free time to visit with me and so we set up a lunch date for Friday at one p.m. by the pool at the Lago Mar.

Shortly before one p.m. on the appointed date, the clouds rolled in and it was clear that outside dinning would not be possible. We both took the initiative and soon we met at the hostess station for the main dining room. It had been five years since we had seen one another, and we exchanged handshakes quickly. Joel had not gained a pound since our last meeting, while I was easily thirty-five pounds heavier. A former lineman on the Lafayette football team, Joel kept in shape primarily by riding his bicycle.

Joel's background included extensive political involvement as well. Early in his career, he served in the Florida State House of Representatives for the district serving Fort Lauderdale. He also was named by three different governors to six different terms as a member of the state's commission on ethics, quite an achievement because he could not serve consecutive terms. Most recently, he has worked as the district director for eleven-term congressman Clay Shaw, a ranking member of the House Ways and Means Committee. Joel also served on the Orange Bowl and Super Bowl committees in years past. He certainly gave me enough information for my class column!

Coincidentally, Friday was also the day I arranged to meet up with Kevin Gilmore, my former coworker from Prudential Bache Securities during 1973 to 1984. In May of 1976, Kevin and my wife Cinnie were both staying at the New York University hospital on 32nd Street and 1st Avenue in New York City. At the age of thirty-four, Kevin was recovering from open heart surgery, while my wife had just delivered our daughter Priscilla via Caesarian section. I made it a point to check up on Kevin whenever I visited the hospital to see my wife, and our friendship grew thereafter.

We met Kevin for dinner at the Bimini Boatyard, and it was great to exchange some old Wall Street stories. When I brandished my traditional underwater camera for a group picture, it reminded Kevin of when he borrowed my yellow Minolta on his rafting trip down the Chatoogaa River in the backwoods of Georgia. The river was the setting for the movie *Deliverance,* which was nominated for an academy award as Best Picture in 1972. While on the trip through the rapids, Kevin's vessel capsized and the borrowed camera spurted overboard and proceeded downstream. Some thirty miles later, when Kevin and his party reached the end of the trip, they were greeted by some of the local "rednecks" who accused the rafters of scaring the fish. Kevin spotted the yellow camera floating on top of the water near their docking point. The pictures were salvaged and the camera lives on to this day.

The day after I saw Kevin in Fort Lauderdale, I felt exhausted, perhaps from the twin social events of the previous day, and/or perhaps from five consecutive days of exercise at the Lago Mar Spa. I suffered from some leg cramps and found walking to be quite strenuous. Raymond and Kelly advised me to go easy on the exercising for a day or two. As the lightning bolts came earlier each day, even swimming was ruled out as an exercise vehicle. Soon, we were locked in the pool bar with our card games and the hours flew by quickly.

In fact, we found ourselves behind schedule as it came time to get ready for dinner. Because I had been freezing up about nine p.m. or so, we decided to cancel our dinner reservation at Charlie's Restaurnat and to dine in the Lago Mar Lounge instead. As I anticipated, I did freeze up and dining so close to "home" made matters easier when it came time to return to our room. While I sat in the walker, Raymond pushed me from the Restaurant to Room 522.

Sunday August 8

As was our customary practice throughout the vacation, I abided by my six a.m. wake-up pill schedule and my wife Cinnie helped me clean up and get ready for the day. Somewhere before seven a.m., I was on my way to the hotel lounge, where coffee was served and editions of the *Sun Sentinel* newspaper were provided. On this particular Sunday morning, Raymond joined me for breakfast and an early attempt at solving the puzzles in the newspaper. They were a bit hard to find, given the massive volume of the Sunday newspaper.

We soon found some puzzles to amuse ourselves and we ordered a sizeable breakfast. Raymond took advantage of the all you can eat Sunday buffet and wolfed down three or four cheese blintzes. I stayed with the traditional orange juice, bacon and scrambled eggs, and coffee.

For months, I had been expressing an interest in possibly moving to Florida. The warm weather was the main attraction. With my Parkinson's factor, the northern winters had become such a hassle. Long pants, outer gear, no golf—all were tough to deal with given my current status. At the age of sixty-six, I figured that there would only be a few more good years left before the PD got a lot worse. Although I loved working with the Lafayette College scene and even hung on to a degree with my Bond Club of NJ affiliation, I felt that a one-floor condo in the Fort Lauderdale area would be a smart move.

In my conversations with Joel Gustafson, he had indicated that some condominiums were located just south of the Lago Mar complex. And so, following our breakfast that Sunday, Raymond and I set out to see what kind of condos were available. I seemed to have more energy than the day before, and so we explored the real estate world adjacent to the Lago Mar properties. Because we were out on a Sunday before nine a.m., our inspection tour would have to be self-directed, without the benefit of a real estate broker.

As we skirted the perimeter of the Lago Mar properties, we came upon a security gate marked "Harbor Estates," and we asked the guard inside if we could inspect any of the units that lay immediately ahead. The guard indicated we would have to come back the next morning (i.e., Monday) sometime after nine a.m. From the exterior, we noticed that most of the units appeared to be two stories and, with a vehicle parked immediately out front, probably inhabited. On our return trip, we passed through the Lago Mar "second lobby" and off in the corner we noticed a Lago Mar Realty sign. Although this office was closed, as anticipated, we were able to pick up some literature on real estate possibilities in the area. Raymond and I felt somewhat optimistic that I could finance the "right spot" if we happened to find it.

At long last, we had a day filled with sunshine, and Raymond and I were determined to get to the beach for a few rays. We had left our deck of Skip-Bo cards in Room 522, and so we doubled back to pick them up. We would do our best not to wake up Cinnie, who frequently slept until after nine a.m.

But as we proceeded down the hall toward Room 522, we could hear a sobbing sound coming from our room. When we reached the door, we were surprised to find it unlatched and the general assistant manager standing inside. My wife, at the point of hysteria, struggled to secure an ice-packed towel around her arm, as swelling started to intensify. When she finally caught her breath and was able to talk, Cinnie explained how she had slipped on the black marble floor between the sink and the toilet. She mentioned a small amount of water had perhaps spilled over from the sink, and this caused her to slip. We calculated that Cinnie's right arm was at worst case broken, probably fractured or sprained, and at best case just bruised. The hotel manager (Paloma) strongly recommended we go to the emergency area of the North Broward Hospital and have the arm x-rayed. She volunteered to make the arrangements for us.

At approximately three p.m., we set out for the emergency room. Although Cinnie didn't have her medical insurance card with her, the Internet verified her coverage by UnitedHealthCare. And so, without any inconvenience, Cinnie was in the queue along with a number of other casualties which had occurred because of Sunday accidents. She was told that the wait would probably be an hour. None of us wanted to leave Cinnie alone, and thus we set up a mini-table and started a Skip-Bo game. Soon, some of the other patients joined in the game. Then, as we heard Cinnie's name called out, Kelly escorted her into the doctor's office, and one of the other patient's support team replaced him in the card game.

Around twenty minutes passed, and Kelly reported that Cinnie had completed the x-ray phase and was just beginning her consultation with the doctor on duty. Kelly rejoined the card game just as his substitute was called into the medical offices.

Around six-twenty p.m., Cinnie and the doctor emerged from the special emergency medical office. Cinnie was attired in a relatively stylish medical smock and her arm was in a cast supported by a sling. We immediately knew this was more than a mere bruised arm. Before we could ask the question, Cinnie volunteered that her arm was fractured. The verdict was not especially good because two of us were now disabled and we were slated to catch a 2:05 p.m. Continental flight the next day. We were indeed fortunate to have Raymond and Kelly to help us get ready.

Not only to get ready, but to help us once we got home in Chatham. Kelly had just completed a major job and was available to help out in New Jersey, and so he volunteered to accompany us home. Raymond had a variety of matters to take care of (i.e., returning the rental car, picking up Kelly's supplies, etc.), and was slated to fly to New Jersey on Friday August 13. In the near term anyway, the wounded Luscombes would be assured of reliable help.

The night before we left for Chatham, Raymond stayed in Room 522 on the pullout sofa bed. Cinnie was under medical instructions not to use her left arm, and so Raymond's responsibility was to help me, if necessary, get up and out of bed, and then lead me to the bathroom. Once I had completed my functions, Raymond would then lead me back to the bed. The slick bathroom floor, as demonstrated by my wife's accident, was nothing to disrespect, and Raymond got the job done, including getting me ready for breakfast and the trip home.

Since Pamona had been so helpful on the day of the incident, we expected the same sort of cooperation from the front desk when we sought help the day of our flight. My wife's only request was for a female helper so she could go to the bathroom and get dressed. Combined, the actions would have required no more than five to seven minutes of one of the cleaning women's time. But the manager for the front desk denied the request and suggested we call 911 instead. Soon, frustrated by the lack of mobility in her right arm and now frustrated by the Lago Mar, Raymond and Cinnie screamed into the two phones in our room that the hotel owed us a "dresser." Finally, one of the women staying at the hotel passed by, sensed the problem, and was glad to help Cinnie with her personal items. Kelly and Raymond packed Cinnie's suitcase. Given the extended aggravation with the Monday staff of the Lago Mar, we were on the move and out the door in record time. We used Raymond's rental car to get us to the Fort Lauderdale-Hollywood International Airport. Earlier in the morning, Raymond had taken Kelly to the airport; Kelly would wait in Newark for our afternoon flight to get in. Heavy over-bookings kept Kelly from joining us on our flight.

Once at the airport, we both used the airline's wheelchair service. We had allowed more than enough time for the security clearance checkpoint, and so were quite early for our 2:05 flight to Newark International Airport. The strategy to arrive early paid some immediate dividends as the agent on duty, spotting our dual wheelchairs, volunteered to move us forward in the flight cabin. We escalated from row 32 to row 8, right at the bulkhead separating coach from first class. The new seats gave us plenty of leg room and ready access to the bathroom. We hoped our luck had changed.

The next thirty days would be a struggle for Cinnie and me. As a professional telemarketer for the Paper Mill Playhouse in Millburn, she would be unable to dial her phone for at least a month. In addition to the potential earnings lost, the prospect of UnitedHealthcare's denial of coverage despite verifying an operational policy on the date of her fall, gave us a persecution complex. We continued to have negative thoughts about the front desk at the Lago Mar. We just couldn't believe their callous attitude twenty-four hours after setting us up with an appointment at the hospital. As the bills from our vacation rolled in, it seemed so disappointing to have such a negative memory of a resort we had always enjoyed. We didn't think we could ever return to the Lago Mar.

Chapter 8

The Columbia University Research Team for Parkinson's Disease

The Neurological Institute
At Columbia University Division of Movement Disorders
710 West 168th Street New York, NY

With the possible exception of some infamous fictional vampires, no one I know likes to give blood! As a part of three different research study groups at the Columbia University's research center for Parkinson's disease, I had a blood sample taken almost every month and periodic checkups relating to the studies.

Prior to participating in these efforts, I never had any problem with technicians taking my blood for physicals and the like. But somehow, in the course of the multiple extractions, the veins in my arms must have developed a second sense of a pending invasion. They seemed to go undercover, and continually frustrated the personnel at Columbia who were trying to monitor my blood while I was experimenting with the new drugs. On numerous occasions, Ann Tam, the technician assigned to my original case study, tried two or three times before succeeding in eking out a minimal amount of my blood. Sometimes, she had to call in Dr. Reina Benabou to get the job done. Dr. Benabu had a rough time as well.

After Ann left Columbia to take a position with a Houston-based firm, Angel Figueroa took over the technical aspects of my case. He too experienced difficulty when withdrawing blood from my veins. On one particular occasion, he called in one of the other technicians, Aida Ocasio, after three unsuccessful punctures, and she concurred that I had rolling veins that slipped away from the needle as it sought a sample of my blood. The team then used one of the veins on the back of my hand, a more painful procedure but one fairly guaranteed to obtain the appropriate amount of blood.

It's not just the personnel at CU. My urologist, Dr. Perry Sartoria, had difficulty when taking blood in his office. He recently apologized for bruising me on both arms! Actually, in retrospect, the Columbia team of Angel and Aida speculated that the large breakfast I consumed before my appointment may have diverted some of my blood supply to my stomach and the digestive process may have slowed down my circulation. Also, my relatively low blood pressure (110/70) meant that my blood supply was flowing slowly through my veins. Angelo weighed me in at 204 pounds, almost forty pounds heavier than I was two years previously. At any rate, blood-taking episodes have basically been an annoyance, but perhaps there is some significance to my experience.

Throughout the tests, my blood pressure (standing up and sitting down) was stable and generally classified as low blood pressure. My pulse seemed normal, and the team seemed satisfied with my EKG.

Actually, the most grueling test required by the research group was when they wanted me to show up for my appointment in New York City in the off position. The rules of the test were that I could take *no* Parkinson's medicine after midnight on the day of my appointment, which was set for nine-thirty a.m. My friend Raymond Monroe stayed at my house that night and helped me get dressed and cleaned up for the ride from Chatham to New York City and the Neurological Institute (upper Manhattan on 168th Street and Broadway). Aware of my discomfort, the team quickly took note of my off condition, called in the top research doctors, and advised me to take my opening salvo of pills for the day around nine-fifty a.m. Normally, I would have taken them at six a.m. and nine a.m. I think I showed the team a representative off condition for their test. I could barely move!

Fortunately, the PD medicines seemed to kick in even faster than normal, and within twenty minutes I was back in the on column.

The team then administered a series of tests and asked several questions about my behavioral pattern. Many of the tests evaluated my coordination, as I followed the nurse's index finger with my own. I crossed my arms and was instructed to stand up without a push from my arms. Once standing, the doctor in charge—either Dr. Waters or Dr. Frucht—tried to pull me down with a strong nudge. This was to test my balance and the likelihood of my falling. I managed to remain standing.

They also tested my memory. At the start of the test, I was asked to remember three words: HOUSE ROAD PHONE. After a passage of about ten minutes and several non-related questions, they asked me to name the three words. I succeeded on this score as well. I had to redraw the framework of a transparent house. They asked me to subtract 7 from 100. Then, I was asked to subtract 7 more, and I responded 86, then 79, then 72, and so forth. They wanted a record of my handwriting, so when asked to write a sentence, I employed the familiar line from typing class: "The quick brown fox jumps over the lazy dog." As always, they asked me about my level of saliva, and my response was that there was nothing unusual about it.

At each visit, the tests were fairly repetitive, and so I could anticipate my response before the technician or doctor could complete the preliminaries. Nonetheless, I am sure they were looking for any *change* in my fundamental condition.

On two separate occasions, I participated in research tests for new drugs designed to mitigate the impact of Parkinson's. Although neither made it to market, the experience of being tended to by the top neurologists in the country who were at the forefront of technology gave me comfort that I was at least proceeding properly in attacking my permanent ailment. It was most disappointing when the second project failed, because this drug (let's just call it Study Group II) had real potential to make life easier for the PD victim. Basically, the drug smoothed over the wearing off periods of Sinemet and as nearly as possible gave the patient a relatively level ride for the day.

Another aspect of the requirements of the study was that I kept a chart of my on and off periods on the days shortly before my official checkup in New York. The researchers were most excited about my chart for this Study Group II medicine. My chart was a straight line of check marks in the on column for a number of the days in question.

However, according to scientists working on the pill, Study Group II apparently produced mineralization in the brains of rats. Presumably, the same was true in humans. So while enjoying the fruits of this pill for most of the summer of 2003, the discomforts of PD returned to my life in full force once the Study Group II was pulled from the testing phase in October 2003.

Part of the test results were intentionally clouded by the placebo effect, which apparently presents an enigma for most Parkinson's research efforts. The placebo pill, which is an imitation that looks and tastes like the one under study but which lacks its potency, is administered via a double-blind trust so that neither the patient nor the doctor knows which type of pill is being tested. Only at the central controls of the test (which I refer to as "The Wizard of Oz") is the actual identity of the type of pill placed on record. In the case of PD drugs, apparently many participants in these studies have reported favorable effects from the use of the placebo drug, which perhaps implies that many Parkinson's problems are psychological in nature.

When I have an appointment with Dr. Waters, she usually includes a trainee or intern in the session. I enjoy hearing her explain my responses to her questions to the neophyte physician. It always seems to me that she maintains a very active schedule, such as meetings with the research staff, lectures, case studies, and appointments with her private clients. Time is a very valuable commodity to Dr. Waters, and so I generally fax her a memo prior to our appointments so as to efficiently update her on my PD condition. She has kept all my memos in a file, and thus she has an ongoing diary of my case. A copy of her book, *Diagnosis and Management of Parkinson's Disease* sits prominently on her desk.

When I ask Dr. Waters to increase the doses of my medicine so as to relieve some of my freeze-ups, if anything, she will recommend a gradual increase in the amount of PD medicine that might be added to my daily menu. She seems to prefer altering the timing or combinations of the various meds while keeping the overall level unchanged. She expresses concern about the resultant dyskinesia from taking more pills. She questions my own management and experimentation, but doesn't expressly prohibit me from such activity.

In my pre-appointment memo for June 21, 2004, I mentioned that the once powerful Sinemet CR pill was possibly slipping in its effectiveness. I posed the following question: Could my lying awake waiting for the pill to "kick in" possibly influence its effectiveness? Actually, the tiny pill used to work better before I wrote about it in this book and it just woke me by surprise! Now, many mornings, I wait for the CR to pop or provide a surge, and nothing happens.

Oddly enough, over the latter part of the time lapse between my two appointments, I noticed a sudden reduction in the number of my severe freeze-ups. Could this be a reaction to the delayed impact of the CR pill? During this phase, I was on almost all day, albeit cautiously, until around six-thirty p.m. As this prolonged on cycle started to slip away, I felt myself drifting into a prolonged off period, and no amount of extra pills corrected the situation. This was modestly disruptive to my schedule for attending evening events such as basketball games, post–golf tournament dinners, and the like. I usually am in bed by ten p.m.

Without any further adjustments to my pill schedule, my on–off cycle seemed to work back to its two-and-a-half to three hour cyclical rotation.

When questioned about brain cell surgery, Dr. Waters' response is that I am a candidate, but not for another six to nine months or so. At the very least, she mentioned waiting until after my daughter's wedding in November 2004. Dr. Melvin Vigman, my original neurologist, has written Dr. Waters recommending the surgery right now!

While at the Institute, you can see broad spectrum of cases of PD. The patients assembled in the waiting room exhibit almost every stage of Parkinson's disease.

In October 2004, I had appointments with both Dr. Waters and Dr. Vigman. The meeting with Dr. Waters was noteworthy because it marked the first time my wife was unable to accompany me to the Institute. In her absence, I conscripted Kelly and Raymond to drive me to the appointment. Because my wife always dropped me off at the emergency ramp, I never actually saw where she parked the car. My advice to Kelly was to drive around and keep parking the car in illegal slots until Raymond and I were done with the appointment. So many cars were illegally parked (mostly double parked) that one more would not make a difference. Kelly abided by my recommendation and kept moving the car from one spot to another. However, in making one of his shifts, he found himself irrevocably locked into the lane leading to the George Washington Bridge and the State of New Jersey. Fortunately, he took the first turn in New Jersey, which circled him around and headed him back to New York. Considering the volume of traffic, the multitude of signs, and his unfamiliarity with the area, Kelly did well to return to the Institute area, where he resumed his weaving from one parking slot to another.

Kelly's plight was compounded by the delay in my appointment. We were early and Dr. Waters was running late, and so our one o'clock turned into a two o'clock. Dr. Waters said I should use my dandruff shampoo. She noticed some white flakes on my shoulders and wanted me to use Desonex whenever I showered. She indicated that dandruff or flaking was common in Parkinson's patients. She wanted me to look good for my daughter's wedding! Also, she inspected my walking and was apparently satisfied. Once again, she was unable to pull me over when I was standing in an open space.

I informed her of my new experiment with the sleeping pills she had prescribed for me almost a year before. I was no longer seeing the men in the white coats, and so on occasion I have been using the prescribed sleeping pills, or Tylenol PM. Instead of tossing and turning all night, and impatiently taking my meds at five-thirty a.m., I frequently sleep until after six a.m. Although I have often had a sluggish start to my day during this experiment, I have noticed an increased energy level as the day wears on.

I also gave Dr. Waters the rundown on my efforts to improve my physical condition through visiting the gym at the Kessler Institute while my wife was undergoing her PT for the arm she fractured while on our Lago Mar vacation. A strong believer in the value of such therapy, Dr. Waters then wrote me out a prescription for another dose of physical therapy.

Finally, as I started on my third research effort, which entailed the open-label study of a new drug, I became interested in the forthcoming World Parkinson's Congress to be held in February 2006 in Washington, D.C. The Congress would include technicians, doctors, researchers, patients, and their families discussing all aspects of the PD phenomenon. We soon discovered that Dr. Waters would be one of the featured speakers. The Conference gave us a new project and we started making preparations almost immediately.

Chapter 9A

The Role of Physical Therapy

Morristown and Moorestown are two distinct communities within the borders of New Jersey. Morristown is located in the northern part of the state and has direct transportation links to New York City. Moorestown is located in the southern portion of the state, near Philadelphia. Both towns have populations of about 16,100. Morristown has a long history dating back to the Revolution, and has a national park featuring George Washington's headquarters. The town's colonial atmosphere and emphasis on history makes it distinctive. Morristown is also a commercial center of sorts, and features the county courthouse for Morris County. Moorestown is a quiet community with a Quaker influence. There are no bars in Moorestown. Morristown in the north has a number of restaurants and pubs. There should be no reason to confuse these two communities.

After my appendix operation in February, everyone was trying to line me up with a physical therapist. Once the wound had healed (a story in itself), my friends and

family were out in the marketplace seeking a PT program that would make my Parkinson's disease more
tolerable. I overheard my friend Raymond Monroe (a
native of Alabama) talking on the phone with a Nova
Care physical therapy group in what I thought was
Morristown. Morristown is less than ten miles away
from us. The clerk for the PT group gave Raymond an
800 number and soon he had us booked for our first
appointment. I had difficulty with directions, however,
as the clerk had given me instructions on how to get to
133 Main Street and I was unaware of any Main Street
in Morristown. Using the Mapquest service on the
computer, I entered the details and somehow the service plotted our drive, with our destination an address
somewhat resembling 133 Main Street. I tried to get
more detail by dialing the Nova Care branch via its
800 number, but the clerk mentioned an unfamiliar in-
tersection. I asked if the Nova unit was near the Dublin
Pub, and she said there were no bars in Morristown.
With these new directions, Mapquest led us to a dead
end in a residential section of Morristown. My wife's
parents were Quakers and she seemed to recall the
Quaker influence in Moorestown. Discouraged by our
lack of achievement, we headed back toward our home
in Chatham.

While traveling from Morristown to Chatham, my
wife remembered that a friend of hers (Alice Burgess)
had had physical therapy at 300 Madison Avenue in
Madison. We decided to make a u-turn and check out
the facilities at that address. We soon discovered
MARA (Morris Area Rehabilitation Association). We
liked what we saw, we used Mrs. Burgess as a reference,
and soon we were scheduled for physical therapy for the

following Friday. The administrator—Edie Gerard—easily opened up our account. When we got home, we verified that the Nova Care office was in Moorestown, not Morristown, and that was that.

Actually, I had taken physical therapy on several occasions in the past. For example, following my back operation in 2000, I undertook extensive PT at the reputable Kessler Institution in West Orange. The facility had gained national recognition when the late Christopher "Superman" Reeve received extensive therapy following his horse-back riding accident. When we applied there in 2003, it appeared they were operating at capacity and they referred us to Nova Care in Livingston. I truly enjoyed the Livingston arrangement, but the corporate entity had a falling out with the local landlord and the entire branch was shut down abruptly in January 2004. For a few weeks, I tried the Nova Care in New Providence, but I felt the set-up lacked charisma, or some other intangible quality. But my appendix attack sharply ended my New Providence connection, and when my doctors gave me another PT prescription, I sought someplace with a little more pizzazz! We had hoped that Nova Care of Morristown (no such place, as we found out) would be the answer, but we wound up in the good hands of MARA of Madison.

My first appointment at MARA involved extensive paperwork and an orientation on how they would approach helping me cope with PD. I told the staff that I wanted to improve my balance and be able to stand up for longer periods of time. I wanted to continue playing golf, not necessarily in championship form, but just playing! I also mentioned that my daughter Alison was getting married in five months and I wanted to be able to escort her down the aisle. Ironically, the wedding reception was slated for the Madison Hotel, almost directly across Madison Avenue from the MARA facility.

After my objectives were outlined, my therapist (Christie) put me through a number of light exercises. She then outlined ten exercises that I could do from my home. I was surprised at how fast the hour went, and it almost seemed exhilarating to do something of a physical nature!

The second trip to 300 Madison Avenue involved a more active session and my therapist for the day (Bhavini Patel) was intent on stretching out the hamstring muscles connecting my legs and ankles, particularly my weak right side. For openers, I tried a ten-minute warm-up cycle on the exercise bike. I was a little annoyed at the seat of the exercise bike, as I kept tilting forward. I like to do a crossword or read a little bit while I bike, but the awkward seat made it necessary to hold on with both hands. Without some sort of diversion, ten minutes can seem like an awfully long time!

After biking, I proceeded to a red matted bed and Bhavini instructed me to lie on my back. She immediately went to work stretching out my legs, starting with my left leg. With my right leg lying flat on the mat, she straightened out the right leg and simultaneously raised my leg toward my chest and took it as far as it would go. She proceeded at a very slow pace and essentially left it up to me as to how far she could go. My threshold for pain was much greater on the left side than my right. She seemed impervious to any moans and groans, and I hoped she would stop soon. I felt her actions were doing me some good, but it sure seemed that she could have done the drill at a slower pace. "No pain, no gain," an expression I learned some fifteen years ago at a Jack LaLane exercise class, crossed my mind as she pursued her course.

A series of other exercises kept me busy until my allotted hour was complete. Bhavini asked me to stand up and when I did, I felt a little light-headed. Her supervisor told me to sit down and she brought me some water. Given my overall inactivity since my appendix operation, I guess my physical condition had slipped more than I thought. I was indeed quite sore, but I would pursue my goals nonetheless.

As I worked on my conditioning at home, I might have injured my right leg when I tried to jump from the low seat of my wheelchair. I was trying to achieve a "hard" landing, thereby breaking up a sustained freeze-up that I was experiencing. I feared trouble lay ahead when I felt my right knee jam upon reaching the ground. The morning after the hard jump, my right leg felt extremely stiff and I had a rough time getting out of bed. Finally, I awakened my wife Cinnie by way of the special alarm that I administer from my bedside. In a matter of seconds, she had me walking toward the bathroom. I felt concern as I felt myself dragging the right foot. The foot itself felt like it was sound asleep, and I was concerned about how I would perform at physical therapy later on that morning.

Before I got into my exercise session, I explained to the PT instructors about my sore right knee. Christi felt the knee and massaged it to hopefully loosen up the joint. She then reduced my number of minutes on the exercise bike from ten to seven. I also stretched out my legs with some wall pushups. For the next exercise, I sat on a colorful beach ball and shot a basketball at a children's net about seven feet off the ground. Now, that was an exercise I really enjoyed, although my shooting percentage resembled that of Shaquille O'Neal, whose foul shooting record hovers around 50 percent. But as soon as I finished with the hoops, I suddenly felt another freeze-up coming on. The therapist offered me some salty peanuts and nuts from a combination raisin mix she had prepared. Visions of my nutritionist and her no salt diet came immediately to mind. At any rate, I took a full dose of my pills (about an hour early) and within about fifteen minutes I was creeping back to normal or the on position.

For my fourth session, I substituted a five iron from my golf bag for my normal cane. I was trying to convey that I was hoping to get my golf game back on track via the PT activities. Christi assured me that the next session, weather permitting, we would go outside and work on my golf swing. Indeed, at session number five, the minute I walked into the therapy site, Christi turned me around and headed me for the front lawn of the 300 Main Street building.

Passersby had several comments, but we smiled and kept on focusing on fundamental golf. She saw somewhat quickly that I had an experienced presence around the golf ball. The basics of keeping one's head down, maintaining a straight left arm, and taking a nice-and-easy pass at the ball—all part of my natural swing.

My main problem, as a Parkinson's victim who had just had his appendix out, was balance. I felt like I was going to fall down if I swung too hard at the ball. I had little or no problems with shorter irons (five iron and below) but was more concerned about the clubs that would give me some distance. Christi then produced two pillows, which she asked me to stand upon. Then I was to swing the golf club. The pillow exercise caused me to focus more on balancing my lower body, and before long I was making more solid contact with the ball. After fifteen minutes of golf, we returned to the gym for some bike riding, stretching, and foul shooting.

After the PT session, I felt terrific. When I arrived home, I called my friend Doug Hobby to see if he wanted to hit some golf balls at the range. Doug is a man of little wasted motion. He said that he would drive, and he would be at my house in ten minutes. I actually told him to make it a little more like thirty. Once at the range, I began to hit the ball more solidly than I had the previous week.

After hitting range balls with Doug, we set out for Sports Authority to buy some golf equipment. I needed some practice or plastic golf balls for my next PT session, while Doug wanted to take advantage of a fifteen-dollar sale of an upscale pull cart. The next day, I spent time hitting plastic golf balls around the yard. The practice was definitely leading to some improvement, although I could feel a pain settling into my back. I worried that this would persist and produce another sleepless night.

Actually, I had minimal expectations for my golfing "comeback," and I certainly didn't expect to see my handicap in the high teens such as it was for most of my pre-Parkinson's lifetime. I was proud of one round, however, which I played at the challenging Canoe Brook South course in Summit.

On October 6, 2002, playing with Wayne Anderson, my host and fellow Class of 1960 member from

Lafayette College, I carded a 98 gross score. The best part about the round was that I registered two straight birdies on the front side par threes. On holes four and seven, I hit the same club—a five iron—about the same distance, 150 yards, and achieved the same results, leaving myself a seven to eight foot putt for a birdie. I still can't believe I made both putts!

Courses such as Canoe Brook and Rock Spring are getting to be too difficult for me. I dropped my membership at Essex County Country Club for the same reason. I had been a member of the Club for almost thirty years, but it seemed that the management of ECCC sought to continually make the course more difficult. Essex County is a great golf course, but I just couldn't take the way it brought me to my knees almost every time I played!

So I now play at a course more accommodating to my Parkinson's-related golf swing. My main venue is the Pinch Brook Golf Club in Florham Park. Pinch Brook is considerably shorter than, say, Canoe Brook South, measuring 4,653 yards from the white tees, versus 6,400 at CB. Pinch Brook has nine par threes, versus five at Canoe Brook. The association of Pinch Brook with the Morris County Park System also makes the cost infinitely more tolerable than a round at a private course such as ECCC or Canoe Brook. For a Parkinson's victim fighting the disease and the ravages of inflation, this makes life just a little bit easier!

Before I knew it, I had used the ten allowable sessions from the first prescription written by my local neurologist Dr. Vigman. I needed a renewal before I could move onto the next phase. I was quite pleased with the progress in my golf game and overall demeanor since working with the MARA staff, and so I encouraged Dr. Vigman to renew the prescripton, which he did.

The first appointment in the second phase of my physical training was a close rerun of the exercises we tried in the opening portion. Ten minutes on the bike, stretches on the pillow with my feet rotating from front to rear, rising and sitting on the oversized beach ball, and smacking a few golf balls on the front lawn of the facility.

Upon returning from outside, Christi asked me where my daughter's wedding would take place, and I informed her that the church was St. Patrick in Chatham. She asked me how long the aisle was, and I had to admit that I didn't know. Then she asked if we were going for a traditional wedding entrance in which the bride stood on the left and the father of the

bride was on the right. I assured Chris that my daughter Alison, the bride-to-be, was a traditionalist. I am not quite so sure about my "contrarian" daughter Priscilla! Regardless, the whole idea that Chris and the staff were going to do their part in making the ceremony a success gave me some satisfaction. Parkinson's and all, they would do their best to see that I was mentally and physically ready to escort Alison in her finest hour. Now that's "custom" PT!

The weather forecast for the final full weekend in July called for extensive thundershowers covering the full time period. Because of the pending storms, for the next session we stayed totally indoors. Chris was really busy since Bhavini had a vacation day; about five patients seemed to be somehow occupying her time. The morning might have represented a warm-up drill for

Chris, because Bhavini would soon be on maternity leave. She instructed me to lie down on the mat and she set me up for an exercise where I raised each leg fifteen times, two repetitions for each side. When she circled back to check on my progress, I was sound asleep. She was in no mood for poorly motivated therapy patients, and she appeared, on the surface at least, to be a bit upset with me. I assured her that the medications and Parkinson's disease were the culprits that produced my narcolepsy. Soon, she had me on my feet doing routines that involved heal-to-toe walking and standing. Chris also introduced me to the treadmill with a five-minute exercise. She asked if I was familiar with the treadmill, and I said I had one in my basement. She asked me the last time I used it, and I responded, "Four years ago!" She encouraged me to reactivate my home machine and work out more often.

One exercise seemed to negatively impact my physical well-being. One of the substitute therapists had me roll my back on a half-cylinder device with a flat bottom. As I attempted to do twenty repetitions, I felt a strange tinge surge through my back and butt. It was reminiscent of the sciatic nerve problems I had experienced some five years prior. Similar exercises had led me to discontinue a program at Bally's Gym three years earlier. I explained to the sub trainer how I felt, and she told me to stop the exercise.

Prior to my next exercise class, I had struggled through a four day case of a sore back. Chris explained that the exercise tool shouldn't have produced that result, but I couldn't deny my discomfort.

Near the end of the second leg of my PT with MARA, my wife and I ventured to Florida for a nine-day vacation. (See chapter entitled "Vacation II.") Anxious to continue my physical exercise program, I set out each day with a routine at the resort's exercise spa. At approximately eight a.m. every day, I vigorously rode the bike and walked the treadmill. As the week wore on, however, I began to feel worse and my Parkinson's freeze-ups seem to intensify.

Shortly after returning home from vacation, I participated in my own self-created Class of 1960 Golf Tournament. As I sought to lengthen out my drives by using my "Big Bertha," I could feel the power swing torque my back. My historically reliable iron swing had turned inconsistent and I began to rely on Bertha. At the finish of the round, I was very sore. The next day, I could hardly move.

A little rest seemed to help me recover from my aches and pains. I did a test run down the aisle at St. Patrick Church, and that seemed quite manageable. At my final session with MARA, Christi had me dancing to a box-like fox trot waltz, yet another pre-wedding preparatory move.

The formal PD program was over. Christi explained to me that I could use the MARA facility as a gym for just forty dollars per month. I planned to sign up as soon as I was feeling a little more strength in my body.

The Kessler Institute for Rehabilitation, West Orange New Jersey

As a young college graduate in the early to mid 1960s, I was a reservist in the New Jersey National Guard, and while en route to my weekend drills at the armory on Pleasant Valley Way in West Orange, New Jersey, I would pass the huge medical facility for Kessler Institute for Rehabilitation. Naively, I wondered if the building housed an investment department or perhaps administered a foundation with the purpose of enhancing the value of the charitable donations made to the institute. Actually, these thoughts were not so far-fetched, because my youthful customer prospecting led to my opening the Clara Maas Building Fund account via the conduit of a third party investment manager.

But some forty years later, my travels would take me to the Kessler Institute as a physical therapy patient with Parkinson's disease. Inside the building, the institute's only visible association with the financial markets was the Bank of America automatic teller machine. The rest of the building was dedicated to in-house and out patient care for those suffering from accidental injuries or from any form of disease. As mentioned earlier, midway through 2004, my wife broke her arm in a fall at the Lago Mar Resort in Fort Lauderdale (for details, see the chapter entitled "Vacation II"), and the doctor prescribed physical therapy at Kessler as part of her healing process. At the same time, coincidentally, Dr. Waters in New York City was prescribing PT for me to make me more agile for my daughter's forthcoming wedding (see the chapters "Wedding Preparations" and the "Day of the Wedding").

However, attempts to simultaneously book our PT times at Kessler were unsuccessful. While my wife obtained an appointment time immediately on submitting her prescription form, my application was put on hold until a therapist became available. I had a chance to witness the therapy process, though, because I dropped into the admissions department every time my wife had her PT. Before moving out to use the exercise equipment in the Kessler gym, I would stop off and subtly remind the admissions officer of my desire to get signed up for therapy. Finally, after being wait-listed for almost the entire time period of my wife's therapy, an opening opened up for me. My appointments would be on Tuesdays and Thursdays from eleven-thirty to twelve-thirty, and would run approximately three weeks depending on their success.

The unwritten motto of punctuality, efficiency, and teamwork seemed to be at the foundation of the institute's operation. In my case, I was initially introduced to two therapists, Kelly and Maureen. By the fourth week of my therapy, I had worked with Allison, Andrea, and Denise in addition to my primary attendants.

Maureen was the "captain" of the team, and she always handled my case between noon and twelve-thirty. The balance of the instructors disappeared at noon for lunch. Thus, if I was to get my full hour's worth of therapy, it was fairly imperative that I get to the session at or before eleven-thirty. Punctuality was much more critical at Kessler than at MARA because of the intricacies of the multiple assignments handled by each therapist. Thus, when I arrived ten or fifteen minutes late for an appointment, I immediately heard about the transgression. Although the remarks of the therapists were couched so as to make it a humorous situation, underneath it all I knew they wanted me to get the message. Be on time!

On one occasion, after I fell during the first snowstorm of 2005, Kelly called me the night before a therapy session to indicate that the neurologist Dr. Frucht from Columbia had given the green light to continue therapy. As we were about to sign off, I assured Kelly that I would be at the therapy session the next morning promptly at eleven-thirty. "That's great," she replied. I was confident I would be on time because Kelly Dodson was my designated driver, and sure enough I pulled into the Kessler rehabilitation room at 11:29 a.m. the next day. Maureen jokingly made a request for some oxygen!

From the standpoint of efficiency, the Kessler therapists were not too fond of my doing crossword puzzles and/or working on my manuscripts while I either waited to be treated or use the various exercise equipment. They would make a point about focus and thinking about one's posture whenever I tried to do something extracurricular.

One of the main objectives of the program was to build my strength. Kelly put me through extensive exercises whereby I stood up from a seated position without providing any thrust from my hands and arms. She exhorted me to use the strength of my lower knees. She constantly yelled out, "Too fast!!!" Kelly was also working on my gait and basic walking structure. Here too, she was constantly telling me to slow down. Andrea, a partner of Kelly's in training from the Philadelphia unit of Kessler, frequently stated that "Momentum is overrated"—another way of saying to take it easy.

As I thought of the therapists' remarks and attitudes, I could take the heat but I wondered if they understood the difficulties facing a PD victim trying to get something accomplished in the off position. On many a night, the only way I make it up the stairs at our house is through relying on the phenomenon of momentum. I have to move very quickly up the stairs and if I slow down along the way, I am apt to freeze up at a very disadvantageous location. When I'm in bed, momentum enables me to get to the bathroom and back, in most cases without assistance, providing I don't linger along the way.

Kelly (often jointly with Andrea) frequently spent a good deal of my session monitoring my walking activity with my rollader (walker). As they walked behind me, I could hear them quietly discussing my case. Their conversation was structured in the medical vocabulary of the times. For example, I could hear them talking how I was pronating my right foot (turning inward while walking) or that the foot exhibited some supination (movement to outward position).

The Brace

Many of the doctors who have examined me have noticed that my right foot actually is a "drop foot." It tends to have little muscle power on its own and can be dragged down with a minimum of pressure even when the doctor asks me to resist the pressure. I can keep my left foot in place, while my right foot simply collapses. When I undertook a minimally invasive back procedure at Morris County Memorial Hospital in Morristown, the physical therapist who was on duty as a requirement for my discharge noticed my drop foot and she recommended a hard plastic brace to help my recovery toward a normal gait.

As I tried to adapt to using the brace, I met with varying opinions as to its ability to help me walk better. Dr. Waters, my neurologist at the Columbia University Neurological Institute, felt the brace had a very favorable impact on my walking appearance. She wanted me to wear the brace all the time. The physical therapists at Nova Care, most notably Jonathan and Christian, thought the brace was not helpful. The physical therapists at MARA thought the brace needed some extra padding so as not to dig into my leg. The physical therapists at Kessler wanted to make an entirely new brace, one which configured with my leg and foot and which would modestly improve my walking stride. On a Thursday afternoon, they set me up with the Brace Clinic.

Parkinson Support Group of Morris County

As a part of my New Year's resolutions, I decided to participate more broadly in the activities of the Morris County Parkinson's Support Group. Ever since she learned of my affliction, my wife had attended monthly meetings of this group. Early on, I had opted to ignore my Parkinson's deficiencies, and so I did not attend any of their functions. Some twelve years or so after discovering my fate, I felt I was forever stuck with PD and ought to see how some of the others my age were coping with the disease.

The first event I attended was the holiday party held shortly after the new year in 2005. We heard some inspiring talks and sang some songs, and the cake was good for desert. Barbara Farrel, spokesperson for the group, announced an exercise class on Wednesday afternoons at the Madison YMCA from one-thirty until two-thirty, and I decided to give that one a try. Much to my surprise, the session was quite intense and I felt that I must be grossly out of shape. The pull-ups and the beach ball squats were a strain on my back, but because of peer pressure I couldn't quit! I was sure glad when they collected the beach balls! Following the exercises, Barbara introduced me to the group as an "accomplished author." I told the group about how I was writing this book and several in the class wanted to see the book when I was done. They also quizzed me on why I had retired from Wall Street prematurely, and I basically told them I was nervous about bungling a big order or causing an error involving a big order. My handwriting had deteriorated to where I could hardly read my own memos shortly after I had taken them!

As these questions were being asked, I could feel my body stiffening up, perhaps as a post exercise reminder but also as a warning to my psyche that a PD freeze-up was next on the agenda. Just then, my wife showed up and I informed the group that she had another meeting and that I would have to leave at that point. I figured that if I left, others would follow; but no such luck. It seemed like they all preferred to stay at the meeting. I felt their collective eyes riveted on me as I clumsily mounted my rollader and made it to the hallway.

The next day, a Thursday, I was slated to take my physical therapy session at Kessler Institute. As I tried to extricate myself from my bed that morning, I found I could barely move. When I did get up and around, I think I hurt everywhere on my body. The thought of going to West Orange and working out for an hour was repulsive. I dialed the reception area at Kessler and left them a message: I was not coming to therapy that day because of illness.

On the following Tuesday, at my regularly slated session of PT at Kessler, I explained to Maureen how I had overdone my exercises at the Madison YMCA, just a day after my activities in West Orange. I guess my body, as I tried to get myself back into physical condition, just wasn't meant to do two- or three-day stints. Maureen concurred and advised me to stay on the Kessler schedule until my prescription ran out and then to join the Madison group. She also suggested a modicum of stretching before heading off to their class.

During the first serious snowstorm of 2005, I took a modest fall on the icy path connecting our front path with the driveway. I hit the frozen ground like a NFL quarterback sliding to avoid a hard hit from a defensive lineman. I almost guided my way to the ground.One of the Kessler Institute's rules is that a patient who falls must report it to his prescribing physician and no therapy can continue until the physician endorses a continuance of the PT sessions. I had to endure a delay when I mentioned my little fall in the snow to my therapists. My doctor was with a patient and phoned back long after my session was over.

I constantly heard Maureen say, "Falling is BAD!" The expression hung permanently in my brain. When I first heard Maureen say that falling is bad, I figured I knew pretty much what she was implying. But then when I witnessed the extensive red tape involved with my little fall, I discovered a deeper meaning to Maureen's warning.

Despite my wife's constantly reminding me to brush my teeth, I am sure that on many nights I just forget. Now I must pay the price in the form of dental bills to Drs. Paetzell and Riva.

Chapter 9B

A Matter of Personal Hygiene

Teeth

Shortly after the New Year holiday, my wife returned from a shopping spree all upset. She could not find the wallet where she kept all her credit cards, a collection that included most major cards and cards for every department store imaginable. Efforts to console her, attempts to retrace her steps, all the psychology in the world failed to neutralize her hysteria. I called the 800 number listed on our jointly held MasterCard and reported it lost or missing. The card had no mysterious activity, but I closed out the card as a precaution. Together, we made about thirty similar phone calls and soon my wife had a wallet of updated credit cards at her disposal.

Compounding the agony of the lost credit cards was the 34–degree rainy weather, which seemed to linger forever in the month of January 2005. My wife was definitely letting the elements get under her skin. Everything and everybody seemed to irritate her. As a gesture of good will, I offered to take her out to dinner at one of our favorite local restaurants, Poor Herbies, in Madison. This being a Friday night, the local restaurant scene would be less crowded than it was on our regularly slated Saturday night. The change in plans seemed to lift her mood, and soon we would be off for Herbies. As she put on all her outergear to face the single-digit weather, my wife reached into her coat pocket and there was the credit card wallet we thought she had lost.

Our intuition about Poor Herbies was correct. When we arrived, plenty of tables were available and soon Dennis (the owner's son) showed us to a prime table. Although the waitress supplied us with menus, we hardly gave them a glance. We were ready to order. My wife's choice was a sirloin steak, medium rare with no seasoning. She reiterated her being allergic to garlic and complemented her main dish with a platter of steamed vegetables. I salivated as I envisioned the marvelous flavor of the highly regarded Poor Herbies steak. However, when I ordered my dinner for the evening, I selected one of the pasta regulars—Baked Rigatoni with Cheese. The rigatoni was my standard purchase. I liked it because it not only tasted great, but also was large enough of a pasta noodle that I could stab it with my fork rather than trying to position it on the fork.

My affection for steak had ended with my association with my new dentist, Dr. Roger Paetzell. My previous dentist, Dr. Sylvester, was satisfactory, but I had to traverse a fifteen- to twenty-step stairway to gain access to his machinery. Once near the top of the stairs, you had to step backward two or three steps as you opened a wide Dutch doorway. Actually, the departure from his office frightened me even more. Given my PD factor, I feared leaving his office full of anesthesia, and negotiating that door and steps to the first floor. As such, when I first retired from Wall Street in 1999, I gradually found myself ignoring Dr. Sylvester and not scheduling my six-month check-ups.

My association with Dr. Paetzell came about when my friend Doug Hobby mentioned to me that he had changed dentists. Doug's dental insurance plan did not cover the majority of the Hobby family's expenses with Dr. Sylvester. And so he sought a reputable dentist that was part of his program. More important, he seemed excited with the positive work ethic of Dr. Paetzell. He cited one particular example of when he was suffering excruciating pain on a Sunday and Dr. Paetzell opened up his office and treated Doug that same day.

When I took a look at Dr. Paetzell's office, I quickly noticed a wheelchair ramp leading from the parking lot to the office's rear entry. Also, we had a lot of common interests, especially sports, and so I signed up for dental duty with Dr. Paetzell.

Ever since I was a boy of six years old, I have had difficulty with my teeth. My first episode involved totally knocking out my front tooth while on a sleigh-riding venture near the mud hole pond a block away from my home in Nutley. Then in my high school years, as an aggressive ice hockey player I took a stick to the mouth, and soon I was without two teeth in the most conspicuous of places. I recall my critical interview with the director of admissions at Lafayette College when I had this huge void in the upper part of my mouth following the loss of the second tooth. The third tooth blew out in a hockey encounter at Sky Top Lodge while on vacation with my parents.

Thus, since the age of twenty-two, I have always had a three-tooth bridge in the upper portion of my mouth. Although hockey accounted for the most cosmetic alteration to my teeth, a multitude of cavities in the rear of my mouth kept the local dentist in a high tax bracket. While conceiving a career path in my early teens, I even thought of the possibility of becoming a dentist. I sure was familiar with the procedures. Nonetheless, my teeth continued to deteriorate. Although I brushed my teeth twice a day, I probably didn't brush them properly. Also, there was a void in my dental coverage when I moved from my hometown to New York City. My dentist in New York was Dr. George Elks, who kept business hours to accommodate Wall Street bond traders. He would be ready in his office to attend to my teeth at seven-thirty a.m. and usually I could be at my desk by eight a.m. I always admired him as a self-made man who had emigrated from Latvia and built a strong career on Wall Street. He listed among his clients many of the heads of Wall Street brokerage firms and also Maurice Stans, commerce secretary in the cabinet of President Nixon.

But Dr. Paetzell was not impressed with the work done by his predecessors. He knew my teeth were in poor condition and needed a lot of work. His first step was to x-ray all my teeth. He fixed one of my defective fillings and I was done for the day. His departing remark was, however, that I would probably have to get a "ton of work" done on my mouth. Indeed, at my next appointment, he had the results of his extensive study of my x-rays, and he easily could see four or five extractions of teeth that just couldn't be repaired and which only acted to catch food. Dr. Paetzell had a general policy of outsourcing recommended extractions, and for this job, used the services of Dr. Richard D. Riva of 201 Main Street in Chatham. If Riva were unavailable, Dr. Gerard Begley took his place. To date, Riva has extracted five teeth.

Dr. Paetzell explored the possibility of replacing the long gone teeth with some false teeth attached by a bridge mechanism. Perhaps this would be a bridge that could be put in and taken out at will. He listed the affected areas as "potentially bridgeable," but was concerned that the bridge would catch food and lead to other problems. His decision was that I should carry on my life with a toothless back of my mouth except for the lower left side.

Very quickly, I found difficulty in chewing sirloin steak or filet mignon. I found myself trying to swallow bigger pieces than I should have, and I certainly could foresee the possibility of a piece of steak getting caught in my throat. Also, I found that potato chips were not so pleasing because the sharp edges tended to rough up my exposed gums. My diet, generally speaking, broke down into seafood (salmon, crab cakes, scallops, etc.) and pasta (pizza, rigatoni, ravioli). I also found I could manage chicken, turkey, and ham.

When I worked on Wall Street, my favorite venue for meeting with clients was the restaurant called Sparks located on 3rd Avenue and 49th Street in Manhattan. For years, the Granite Bank of Keene, New Hampshire would co-sponsor a dinner whereby their principal officers and directors met with various members of the Wall Street community. Prior to the event, we all talked about how much we looked forward to a steak from Sparks! Hardly anyone strayed from the menu. We must have ordered twenty sirloin steaks, medium rare! It was unmanly to order anything but steak! I have not been back to Sparks since Dr. Riva pulled all my back teeth.

As a Parkinson's patient, I probably have difficulty brushing my teeth because the traditional times of day for brushing are when I am in the off position. I typically struggle in the morning to simply get dressed and ready for breakfast. Generally speaking, I return to the upstairs bathroom between nine-thirty and ten a.m. and take care of my teeth then. Sometimes I get busy and just plain forget to return to the toothbrush area, and so I skip brushing. Despite my wife's constantly reminding me to brush my teeth, I am sure that on many nights I just forget. Now I must pay the price in the form of dental bills to Drs. Paetzell and Riva.

Prostate

Prostate cancer is very prevalent among men over fifty years old. I discovered my prostate problem when I had a back operation in the fall of 1999.

Immediately after surgery at Morristown Memorial Hospital, I had difficulty urinating. In the middle of the night, my pain from feeling my bladder urging me to go continued without relief and so the night nurse called in Dr. Perry Suteria. He immediately placed me "on the bag," and that relieved the pressure. For the long term, he suggested I make an appointment at his office to check out my PSA. When those tests were back, my PSA registered a relatively high 4.20. Dr. Suteria was concerned but not alarmed. He prescribed two medications, which I take to this day: Proscar and Flomax. Subsequently, my PSA has dropped to 1.2 + and is theoretically out of the danger zone.

At the start of 2005, I was urinating frequently in the middle of the night. I mentioned the situation to the urologist, and he just said, "That's too bad!" It actually helped that he wasn't concerned, and I started to sleep for longer stretches. Also, I started to sleep with a flat pillow between my legs. This solution seemed to limit the friction between my legs and toned down any bladder stimulation. The pillow helped when I got out of bed. The rectangular-shaped pillow, properly wedged under my top sheet, could organize the sheets in a straight line and facilitate returning to bed.

Feet

My feet are on the big side. I wear a size 11.5 D shoe. I have had few problems with the likes of athlete's foot. A bone spur in my left heel seemed to self-correct a few years ago.

The problem with my feet is that the nails are very thick, almost metallic. They are backed by a hardened callous substance. Ordinary clippers or pedicure scissors are ineffective in trimming the tips of my nails. Left unattended, as you would expect, they just grow and grow. They sometimes get tangled up in my socks or make it difficult to put on socks. When I wake up in the night and proceed to the bathroom in my bare feet, sometimes my toes get caught in the carpeting. This may stall me just long enough so I lose my momentum or rhythm. Any time of day, if I take a sudden turn while I'm walking, my toes catch in the carpet.

Pedicurists at local salons have tried to trim these pegs of steel. Some have refused to take an appointment with me until I see a professional podiatrist. I actually dislike going to get a pedicure. Snipping of my toenails typically entails some pain. The pedicurist must route the clippers between the nail and the substance lying between my toe and nail. Once completed, my nails feel very sore.

To make matters worse, the attendant will customarily stretch out my leg while she works on my foot. When she does this, and actually holds the leg in this position for some time, she seems to reactivate some dormant muscles.

Feet II: The Brace Controversy

Up until the end of 2004, depending on my mood, I used to wear a hard plastic brace on my right foot and ankle. The brace was an enigma. Among my various advisors, some said the brace was helpful to me, while others weren't so sure. Dr. Cheryl Waters, who thought she may have even designed the brace, is the most supportive of me using the brace. Physical therapists at the old Livingston facility did not favor the brace, nor did Kelly from the PT staff at Kessler. To me, the brace felt fine and enabled me to walk more consistently without any assistance. It just added to the excess baggage that I had to carry every day.

Kelly at Kessler seemed quite certain that the brace would only provide minimal improvement. In her eyes, it was not snug enough to my right toenails. She also disliked the way the brace dug into my upper right shin. Kelly perhaps would have favored a brace designed by Kessler's own brace unit.

Upon further self-analysis, I found that the brace was a mixed blessing. While I was walking along, I found the brace gave my drop foot extra support. People told me my walking style looked more natural. On the other hand, it took a fair amount of extra energy to get the brace on properly in the morning. Additionally, the sharp edge of the outer wall of the brace did dig into my shin. Lastly, I found wearing the brace made my off periods last longer. If it would help the on periods stay around longer, I would wear the brace 24/7!

Sometimes removal of the brace acts as a stimulant to helping me snap out of one of my rigid periods. The same can happen if I take off my socks or if I start some typing. These maneuvers are designed to give me some momentum for momentum's sake! Oddly enough, they do seem to work.

Whereas the physical therapists at Kessler were jammed by their tight schedule, the Kessler doctors who assessed my foot for a new cast were quite relaxed and running about twenty minutes behind schedule when I came in for my appointment. They allow for a revolving door of patients, and they take clients as they arrive. A group of five doctors and medical personnel assess the brace candidate's needs.

In a matter of five to ten minutes, the medical team decided that a custom-fitted brace would help me walk better and more comfortably. In no time, the team had me shuffled off to the prosthetics lab and the medical assistant (I believe his name was Gil) quickly had my leg in a formative cast. Once the cast was dry, he scissored it open and said the finished product would be ready in two weeks. It was easy to tell that Gil took great pride in his work.

Based on the preliminary testing of my foot with a wrapped ace bandage elevating my middle three toes, I was somewhat optimistic about the effectiveness of the brace. I was overdue for something positive to happen to improve my balance and walking posture. The doctors at Kessler even mentioned my return to the golf course.

Like clockwork, the new and improved brace was ready for me two weeks later. I was the second person on line in the first-come-first-served system used by the brace clinic team. Within minutes, I was summoned into the office. The main doctor quickly showed me the brace and moved to put it on my leg. As I took my first few steps in front of the team of doctors and other medically attired personnel, they were unanimous in approving its impact. There was no doubt in their collective minds: The new brace helped me walk a lot better.

"How does it feel?" asked the doctor in charge.

I mentioned that it seemed a bit snug and applied extra pressure around my arch. He replied that the arch would eventually fold into place in a few days.

I could hardly wait to walk back to the physical therapy area to show Maureen and Kelly the results of their efforts. As I made my way, I passed Gil—the artist who created the brace—and he asked me how it felt. I could tell by the look in his eye that he knew my gait had instantly improved.

Maureen and Kelly also seemed to endorse the brace, and they suggested wearing higher socks to cover the top of the unit. They also advised working my leg as hard as possible by using the exercise gym at the Kessler Institute.

From a longer-term perspective, it was too early in the game to judge the impact on my life. For sure, the day at Kessler left me with a positive attitude.

*No one was shy when it came to asking for money from
the cash fund. They all praised my handwriting on
checks, but claimed they couldn't read my messages on
non-monetary matters.*

Chapter 10A

Wedding Preparations

When Erik B. Swift privately asked permission to
marry my daughter Alison, I was extremely excited. Erik had made a special trip to our house on the
pretext of helping with some holiday decorations, and
so the timing caught me by surprise. He instructed me
to keep his intentions a secret until he actually popped
the question to Alison. After recovering from the initial
excitement, Erik and I shook hands and exchanged a big
hug, and we started to discuss some of the basic details
about the wedding itself. We would get more focused
once Erik had officially asked Alison and she accepted.

After Erik left the house and I had a chance to think
about the significance of his proposal, I started to envision
my own role in the festivities. Situations like walking down
the aisle and dancing at the reception immediately came to
mind. Although my neurologist Dr. Waters had always
said that I could add some extra pills, particularly Sinemet,
to ensure a more "normal performance," I thought about
the times when the bonus pill technique hadn't brought the
desired results within the desired time frame.

Erik's master plan was to make his proposal on their winter vacation in Cancun over the New Year's holiday. The specific site was slated to be atop one of the Egyptian-style pyramids at Chickeniatsu, within the Mayan complex located about an hour or two from Cancun itself. When Alison complained of dizziness as she attempted to climb the difficult stairs of the pyramid, the pending ceremony was rescheduled for sea level. With both feet on the ground, her response to Erik's question was a resounding "Yes!"

When Erik and Alison returned from vacation, an ad hoc committee was established to make preparations for the wedding. Leadership of the committee was quickly assumed by Alison, the chairperson, with her mother being a nearby challenger, perhaps wearing the title of vice chairman. My future son-in-law Erik and his parents would have token votes and act as advisors. My role would be that of chief financial officer. By nature, the committee structure innately created some sources of conflict between Alison and her mother. The rest of us, suffice it to say, were along for the ride.

My somewhat limited role was partially in recognition of my Parkinson's condition. The tremors or rigidities associated with the off periods of PD tend to intensify when I'm under a lot of pressure. Therefore, my number of productive hours may be severely limited during the day. As such, I was initially excluded from a lot of the detail work associated with planning the Swift–Luscombe wedding. My ability to take down phone messages and re-read them to their intended recipient was just not reliable. Also, I would flat out forget to give the person the message. In order to stay current, I created my own shadow file as a back-up to the organizational efforts of Alison and my wife.

No one was shy when it came to asking for money from the cash fund. They all praised my handwriting on checks, but claimed they couldn't tread my messages on non-monetary matters.

Although I had known Erik for almost five years, I was unaware of any strong religious affiliations with either a specific Protestant sect or the Catholic Church. I should have deduced his Catholic connection since I knew he had attended Christian Brothers Academy, a prominent Catholic prep school located in Lincroft, New Jersey. To the extent I followed high school athletics in New Jersey, I was aware that CBA was a continuous contender in football, basketball, and track within the parochial ranks of the state.

My daughter Alison was totally unattached religiously. I recall coaching her with her Elon University undergraduate course covering the Protestant Reformation. On a particularly hot and sunny day in her junior year, Alison decided to cut religion class and work on her tan. Unfortunately, the spot where she chose to sunbathe was in full view of the religion professor and the balance of her classmates. Ten years later, when the site of the church for the wedding arose, Alison deferred to Erik's Catholicism. Quickly, the decision was made to have the wedding at St. Patrick Church, which was located less than a mile from our house in Chatham.

My initial thoughts on the location of the reception: either the Madison Hotel or the Morris County Country Club, ironically both located within a mile of one another in Convent Station. Both possibilities were satisfactory in my initial discussions with Erik, and so I reflected my suggestions to the decision makers, Alison and my wife.

Over the years, since moving to the Morris County area in 1967, we had often dined at Rod's Restaurant (currently attached to the Madison Hotel), and we knew the food to be excellent. Morris County Country Club was a beautiful location, rich in history, and offered an element of prestige to the occasion. The hotel could accommodate a slightly larger crowd, while the Club maxed out at 200 people. Although lodging arrangements would be quite convenient if we chose the club, Madison Hotel's on site facilities gave it an obvious advantage. I set up interviews with the appropriate contact people at both locations, and the Alison–Cinnie team subsequently met with both institutions. Other clubs and restaurants were considered and visited, but I believe the two finalists were the Madison Hotel and the Morris County Country Club.

Soon, the decision was made and the Madison Hotel was named as the site for Erik and Alison's wedding reception. I was instructed to send a $100 deposit to hold the reservation for the date of November 13, 2004, which at the time was some nine months away. A much larger check representing 10 percent of the estimated bill would be required in June. Considering the volatility of the stock market and given the length of time to run to the wedding date, I sold two stocks (Caterpillar Tractor and Chittendon Trust of Vermont) and escrowed the proceeds to hopefully cover the full cost of the event. The process and the dollar amounts reminded me of planning for college tuitions for my daughters in the early 1990s.

The activities relating to the wedding over this eleven-month span were easily handled by the Alison and Cinnie team. My main trauma, initially, was that I would miss the Lafayette College–Holy Cross home football game. At least we skirted the November 20 match-up with archrival Lehigh. In any case, I was less than excited about the prospects for Lafayette's football team. Coming off of a 5–6 losing record in 2003 and facing seven road games in 2004, it looked like another disappointing season for my beloved Leopards. As I thought ahead, I would be missing just another game if I couldn't attend the Holy Cross contest because of the wedding.

The committee's first stop was Priscilla of Boston, a wedding dress store located in Short Hills. Alison's younger sister Priscilla had just moved from Boston to Washington, D.C. Only two weeks after the actual engagement, the various bridesmaid dresses and the wedding gown were decided in just one visit to the wedding dress store. I figured there would be more comparison shopping for such a critical item, but I guess the committee had a strong conviction as to what was needed.

The next activity was the engagement party held in mid-January at the popular restaurant in Hoboken known as Franky and Johnny's. For this event, I was selected to serve on the sub-committee for decorations, a low pressure job that entailed my contacting the bookstores of Purdue University and Elon University, Erik and Alison's respective alma maters, and purchasing some colorful triangular shaped pennants to help adorn the premises. The bookstores were accommodating and the banners arrived in plenty of time for the party. My wife was concerned that the colors on the banners were not the true colors of the respective universities. We also argued over the meaningless configuration of a Boilermaker, the Purdue official mascot. I assured her that the colors were reflective of my understanding of the college colors. The potential clashing of the banners with the flowers was a minor problem as far as I was concerned.

More important, the party was our first meeting with John and Nancy Swift, Erik's parents, and we seemed to get along with one another very well. As the party drew to a close, I had a modest freeze-up and had to be pushed up to the car in my walker. I wished I could have made it all the way, but PD has a mind of its own.

As I thought of the wedding date in November 2004, I continuously felt some anxiety when I tried to visualize what sort of physical condition I would be in for the event. Although my daughter would be the featured attraction, I knew I would be one of the first ones up as I escorted her down the aisle to the musical notes of *Here Comes the Bride* or perhaps Purcell's *Trumpet Solo*. I didn't want to use a cane or a walker in the church, and I wondered how far my Parkinson's might degenerate over the span of Erik and Alison's somewhat lengthy engagement. Nonetheless, I knew the emotional high concurrent with hearing the beginning of the bridal march of my own daughter would be intense to say the least. As mentioned in the physical therapy chapter, I did a few practice runs at the St. Pats Church and these were fine.

I also thought ahead to the reception. I used to relish parties and weddings, but with PD, I seem to wear out for the day about nine-thirty or ten p.m. Hopefully,

I would be able to condition myself to last a couple of extra hours. Fortunately, we booked the Madison Hotel for the reception, and my wife and I would have a room nearby, right on the premises.

Alison and Erik lined up my tuxedo and other fancy attachments at the Tux Shop in Hoboken. On September 29, I got myself fitted. My weight and physique continued to be an embarrassment for me. People who mentioned that I looked good were trying to boost my morale or elevate my low self-esteem, or so I felt. For the sake of appearances, I kept up a good front. I knew, for Alison and Erik's benefit, I had to be strong. "The Show Must Go On!" was my motto, and I would keep plugging away as best I could.

I knew that a lot of organizational efforts were taking place, and occasionally my input was sought. I suggested that our family limo service, the ever-faithful Phil, should be used for transporting the wedding party between the wedding and the reception. But Alison wanted a real professional team to produce some eye-catching limos, and so I was overruled. His was a one-car service, and he could have outsourced the order, but I think Phil understood. The thought came to mind that perhaps Phil could play a different role and act as security for our house while the various ceremonies were taking place on November 13. With a multitude of presents being stored at our unattended household, it behooved us to set up a security system to stand guard. Perhaps Phil was our man!

As it turned out, our faithful friend Vin Morris stayed at our home during the ceremony and my friend Raymond, who took over the night shift, relieved him. Phil was on tap for rides to the airport, most important, the pickup of the bride and groom at five-fifteen on Monday morning, to convey them to Newark Airport for their flight to Hawaii.

The official invitations to the wedding were to be printed as elegantly as possible. Each invitee would receive:

- A formal invitation to the wedding
- A formal invitation to the reception
- A notice of availability of hotel rooms for out-of-town guests
- Directions to the wedding and reception
- A response card, simply stating "accepts" or "declines"
- A self-addressed envelope to our house

The packet contained at least two layers of tissue to protect its contents. The postage per invitee was $0.60, requiring an extra 23-cent stamp atop the standard 37-cent stamp.

The design of the invitations was classic Tiffany script. Alison and her mother were in basic accord with the invitation format. My responsibility was simply to write up directions for people coming from various locations.

The internal conflicts that tended to activate my Parkinson's neuroses were mostly associated with the invitation list. Both families were excited about the wedding and wanted to invite as many guests as possible to celebrate the joyous occasion. The seating capacity of the Madison Hotel would limit us to approximately 250–275 invitees. We expected a fallout of about 20 percent and therefore an anticipated reception crowd of 200–225 people.

My closest friends related to my Lafayette College experience and I initially suggested some seven couples—17 people total. In addition, my wife wanted me to include three more couples, and I indicated that it was time to draw the line. She said she felt uncomfortable attending football games and talking about the wedding without everyone in my group being invited. She also wanted to include many of her coworkers, high school friends, and former neighbors of ours who we hadn't seen for years. It seemed that everyone who called the house or who she encountered while walking the dog, or the person bagging her groceries at the Kings Market—everyone was invited to the wedding. The relatives for the Luscombe and the Swift families contributed some fairly sizeable representations, while Cinnie's Baldwin family was initially only represented by her brother John. Alison and Erik were both very popular and had many friends they hoped would attend the wedding.

And so we all drew up lists of potential invitees, putting them on the "A" list or the "B" list. The B list would be activated if the ratio of declines started to exceed 20 percent. Cinnie continued to lobby for her B list while the rest of us seemed supportive of the A list as suggested. Once the invitations were in the mail a few weeks, and as soon as we had a better sense of how many people would be coming, then we could start drawing on some B list names to accommodate any shortfall. The deadline for the invitees to return their responses was October 16. About October 11, we activated a portion of the B list.

During the first few weeks of October, I experimented with having a few glasses of chardonnay when thrust into social situations. I found the wine had the effect of reducing my inhibitions about meeting people and visiting old friends. Homecoming Weekend at Lafayette provided the testing ground for my new policy. The opening event was the Marquis Society reception. I ordered my wine and then positioned my walker right next to the sign-in desk, where all the participants would pick up their name tags. Anyone I knew had to pass this point, and I recall flagging down many old friends.

The only drawback to my wine-stimulated personality was that I couldn't keep my hand steady. As my conversations gathered momentum, the wine was shaking and starting to spill over the top of the tapered glass. I had wine drops all over my slacks, my shirt and tie, and my sports jacket. The same result occurred when I accepted an hors d'oeuvres from the roving waiters.

Fortunately, I was only signed up for the reception portion of the program. When the clock struck seven p.m., I was like Cinderella as I quickly made my way to the exit while the rest of the guests filed into the dining room. The ever-faithful Raymond was waiting for me in my car just outside the rear door to Marquis Dining Hall.

The week of October 17–24 was indeed hectic for all of us. October 23 was the date of the major bridal shower to be held at my house in Chatham. The pressure was on my wife to organize the house so that it could gracefully accommodate close to forty women. Folding chairs from the garage, the attic, and the basement were resurrected for the occasion. All closets located on or about the first floor had to be emptied and stocked with hangers for the guests' coats. The phone rang all week long as guests called to inquire as to what they might bring to the shower. My wife was somewhat hyperactive as she worked on three (or more) recipes for hors d'oeuvres. The Chatham Mens Club was treated to a week-long sampling of Cinnie's pinwheels, cheese puffs, crab meat dip on a cracker, drunken hot dogs (hot dogs in a bourbon sauce), and more. She also created a rum-daiquiri punch that she tested on my willing friends. Café Beethoven was consigned to provide lunch for the guests once the ladies had worked their way through the preliminaries.

The shower's honoree, Alison, was supposedly unaware of the preliminaries involved with this event. She did, however, have many questions about why we needed the carpets and drapes shampooed, why we were having the interior and exterior of the house painted, and so forth. Keeping the shower a secret was a major effort in itself. We were importing Priscilla from her Arlington, Virginia home, and we slipped her in on the day before the shower.

While the ladies had a great time at the shower, I was off on an excursion to Penn State University, as covered in the "Project Iowa" section of the "Road Trips!!!" chapter. We picked the perfect weekend to be away from the house!

Throughout October, our front door was busy receiving packages from the United Parcel Service. The responsibility of opening these packages rested with my wife and me. The job sounds easy enough on paper, but in reality we piled up an immense amount of cardboard to be recycled, as required by local law. Worse than the cardboard were the Styrofoam gizmos that cushioned each package. These one-inch long objects had to be separately packaged inside an authorized green bag, otherwise the town would not pick them up. These gizmos were exceedingly difficult to control. Efforts to quickly dump them into a green bag resulted in most of them landing on the floor. They all had an annoying sticky substance that made them cling to the carpet. I finally devised a contraption to hold the bag open as I eased the contents into its inner chamber. For such a busy person with a limited amount of available time, the whole process seemed very non-productive.

Throughout the engagement period I kept wondering how I would handle the events of the wedding date itself. A lot of activities were planned and I was concerned about how long my body would endure on November 13, 2004. My major responsibility was to see that the Madison Hotel was paid for the reception and that the appropriate gratuities were bestowed on the personnel involved with the affair. Tim McHale headed up the crew that ran the reception, and my daughter Alison and I were to meet with him two days before the reception to pre-settle these issues. With respect to these matters, I received some advice from Joe and Gary Sluck, two younger alumni from Lafayette College. Both had worked at the Madison Hotel and also had their wedding receptions there, with Joe's being fairly recent.

The other concern I had was staying up until midnight or one o'clock in the morning. Whenever I tested staying up late, I could barely make it past ten p.m. Oddly enough, *Monday Night Football* gave me the test I was looking for.

Every fall, for at least fourteen years, Ken Thompson and I attend the Miami Dolphins–New York Jets football game at the Meadowlands Stadium (a.k.a. Giants Stadium) and quite often the National Football League has this game highlighted as one of the sixteen games they present on *Monday Night Football*. The negative factor of *MNF* is that the games begin at nine p.m. and usually end close to one o'clock in the morning. For this year, however, I had discouraged Ken from expecting me to participate. But Ken wanted to sustain the tradition, and in lieu of seeing the game in person, he suggested we watch the contest at a sports bar such as O'Reilly's in Maplewood or Hooters on Route 22 in Union. We calculated that halftime would occur about ten-thirty p.m., and we could either watch the second half at the pub or proceed to my house and I could see how late I could remain on.

We decided to go to O'Reilly's and we were joined by Kelly and Raymond, also members of the Chatham Mens Club and avid football fans. Unbeknownst to us, O'Reilly's had been totally remodeled and actually resembled a sleek New York bar. We ordered some drinks and dinner, and were all set by kick-off time. As one of the few Dolphin fans in the pub, Ken was outnumbered three-to-one. Two late scores in the first half, including a 51–yard field goal with just :01 left on the clock, gave the Jets a 17–7 lead at the intermission. I felt fine, but was skeptical as to how long I could make it, so Ken and I left for my house where I could stay up as long as possible, and then simply roll into bed! We watched the game in my living room, and I felt on until about eleven-fifteen p.m. At that point, the game began to evolve into a strictly one-sided affair in favor of the Jets, so I mentioned to Ken that it was time for me to go to bed.

My late night was accomplished with one bonus pill taken about eight p.m. (corba doba lopa doba) in the evening. The evening was a successful tune-up for the wedding reception just twelve days away! Perhaps all I needed was one or two more pills and I could go the distance!

On the Tuesday before the wedding, I started another session of physical therapy, this time returning to the active facilities of the Kessler Institute in West Orange, as covered in Chapter 9A. I had hoped to resume PT several weeks prior, but the therapists at Kessler were all carrying a full caseload. I was thankful to get two sessions under my belt before the wedding. I was counting on my conditioning program to help me walk down the aisle on the wedding date.

Following my orientation with my assigned therapists, Kelly and Maureen, I embarked on a program to *strengthen* my muscles and to enhance my balance. I mentioned to Kelly and Maureen my objective of performing well at the wedding just four days away. During the second session, just fifty-one hours before the church ceremony when I would march down the aisle alongside my daughter Alison, Maureen gave me a number of leg exercises to perform. As I approached the limits of exhaustion, I informed her that I didn't want to overdo things before the wedding. When she was reminded of the impending blessed event, she told me to stop right away. Maureen seemed to have overall confidence in my ability to do all the exercises. But she didn't want to destroy me before the official ceremony.

At home, tensions were running high throughout the week. My wife had a ton of chores lined up for Raymond, Kelly, and me. The guys also wanted to secure an appropriate wedding gift, and they were a little late in trying to use the bridal registry at three stores and finally settled on a gift from Macy's.

The day before the wedding, we had near-freezing rain, highway traffic was in gridlock, and airport delays were reported everywhere on the map. In short, the weather was just horrible everywhere in the Northeast. Raymond, Kelly, and I rushed through the various chores assigned to us, which included a stop at Broccalini's Restaurant to deliver the wine and beer for the impending rehearsal dinner. We then checked into the Madison Hotel fairly early, around three p.m. We wanted to secure a good location vis-à-vis the reception, and the hotel management accommodated us with a first floor room. Also, since my wife would be occupying the room the following night, it was important that the windows opened.

Chapter 10B

The Wedding Date

The Madison Hotel/Wedding Central
Convent Station, New Jersey
November 13, 2004

A slight dusting of snow partially covered the cars in the Madison Hotel parking lot early on the morning of November 13, the date of the Luscombe–Swift wedding. Brilliant sunshine radiated through a modicum of clouds and made the weather seem a touch warmer than the 27 degrees posted on the thermometer. As the day wore on, the temperature approached a comfortable 50 degrees. The day was surely a pleasant and unexpected change from the day before, which basically had been wall-to-wall rain. Indeed, for the month of November, it was a near perfect day.

I awoke about five-thirty a.m. and I immediately thought of my gimpy legs and how I would fare on the walk down the aisle with my daughter at my side. I had practiced the walk a couple of times, and had actually done a dry run with my daughter the night before at the rehearsal. In each case, I had negotiated the short walk without difficulty. Still, the pending exercise would dominate my thoughts throughout the day. I had a cane

235

and my walker at the ready, but I was determined not to use either.

Lacking any official responsibilities, my objective for the morning was simply to keep busy and not get nervous about my role in the ceremony. First I chatted with Patti Ellingham, whose husband worked with me in the late 1960s at Halsey Stuart & Co. We enjoyed some coffee and buns together about seven a.m. Later in the morning, Kelly and Raymond proposed we have a game of Skip-Bo in the hotel lobby. By playing cards out in the open, I could accommodate one of my wife's requests, which was to keep an eye out for my ninety-three-year-old Uncle Willie. Uncle Willie was a native of Coronado, California (near San Diego) and had captained a mine sweeper during World War II. Actually, we encountered several of the guests in the lobby and the atmosphere at the continental breakfast was like a tranquilizer to me. Before I knew it, the clock approached noon and it was time for us to clean up and change into our tuxedos.

Back in Room 109, we hurriedly unpacked our respective tuxedo from their plastic cargo bags. Raymond helped me extract the contents of my bag, and gradually we had cuff links, studs, black cummerbund, and strap-on bow tie locked into place. I opted to forgo the shoes provided by the rental agency. They fit perfectly and looked marvelous, but they were extremely slippery. Given my delicate balance, I decided to wear a new pair of solid black sneakers.

We were trying to abide by the official schedule, as determined by the professional photographer for the wedding. We interpreted that the schedule required us to report to the house in Chatham around one p.m. But when we arrived at the house, a form of organized chaos prevailed as we witnessed the six bridesmaids attired in full-length cranberry red dresses and working vigorously on their appearance. Each of the young ladies sported a distinctly combed hairdo and carried a cocktail consisting of equal parts of orange juice and champagne. The potent mixture (a mimosa) partially explained the joviality of the group. I was immediately offered a glass of this joy juice, but after one sip I decided I had better maintain my equilibrium for the ceremony. Although I wanted to be sociable, even more I wanted to have my Parkinson's pills working their hardest as the three o'clock wedding hour approached. To avoid the temptation of the partying bridesmaids, Raymond and I headed back to the Madison Hotel because we had about an hour before the photographer wanted me in some of the photos.

As it was a Saturday in the fall, we decided to pass the time by watching the early session of college football games on TV. We also had interest in following the line-score of the Lafayette versus Holy Cross game. This short diversion was accomplished at Rod's Bar at the hotel. We were barely seated, when an entourage of ushers and groom Erik Swift joined us. Like their bridesmaid counterparts, they too were enjoying a mid-afternoon cocktail session, which I believe consisted mostly of beers. I ordered a chardonnay from the bartender, but only had a few sips. The hour allotted to football passed quickly, and soon we were on the final countdown to the wedding. We said good-bye to the male portion of the wedding party, and soon we were on our way back to the house in Chatham.

About two-fifteen p.m., I took an extra carbidopa pill (25 mg/100mg) as a precaution against freezing up during my walk down the aisle.

Raymond was scheduled to join Kelly as an official greeter at St. Patrick Church at two p.m., and so he dropped me off at the house in Chatham and sped off to his assignment. He also took along my walker, which he strategically placed in the rear lobby of the church near where the recession would commence.

Meanwhile, a short stint of photographs with the bride (my daughter Alison), the maid of honor (my daughter Priscilla), and my wife Cinnie took place in the front yard. At two-thirty p.m., the stretch limo arrived and the bridesmaids cheered as we prepared to move out to the wedding ceremony.

As the crow flies, St. Patrick Church is a mere six blocks from our house. But the limo driver—given the length of his vehicle—had to take a somewhat circuitous route to the church. On our first foray, we arrived fifteen minutes early and so we elected to drive around the block. My wife Cinnie, who rarely is on time for any event, was in the limo and was technically fifteen minutes early for the ceremony.

An element of anxiety entered my mind as I sat somewhat awkwardly in the limo. Ten minutes sitting in the wrong position could lead to a freeze-up. As I squirmed and moved my upper body, my daughter sensed my concern and soon she ordered the driver to drop us all off. When I worked my way out of the relatively narrow passageway, I was sure glad to feel the solid earth below my feet. Soon I was bounding up the stairs (with the assistance of a railing) toward the lobby of the church. I quickly spotted my walker and sat down where I thought the procession would line up. My legs felt good and active. The eleven months of waiting for this moment were about to end. For what my wife had labeled "The Broadway Production," it was showtime and I would soon be on stage.

Suddenly, I spotted my boyhood friend, now a Catholic priest, Father Lewis Papera. I stood up from my walker and shook his hand, and then quickly we engaged in a huge hug. He was in full garb and would assist Father Hines in conducting the wedding ceremony. When I spotted Father Lew, my whole body swelled with emotion. It was as if my entire life was being tied together.

The groom's younger brother Michael, a six foot, four inch airline pilot, was the usher who seated my wife, which signaled to all that the ceremony was about to start. The remaining ushers moved into position, coming down the left aisle then crossing over to the right side of the altar. Then, in single file, the bridesmaids slowly made their way toward the altar. I remained sitting until the last bridesmaid (the maid of honor, my daughter Priscilla) started her stroll down the aisle. I then rose and took my place by the side of the bride, my daughter Alison.

The organist gave us the go ahead by playing the opening notes of the processional, *Canon in D Proceeded by Trumpet Voluntaire.* Without hesitation, Alison and I, arm in arm, were in the church proper on full display in front of more than 200 wedding guests. Stephanie Serwatka, a bridesmaid and a lifelong friend of Alison's, remarked that the only other time she saw the church as full was at Christmastime. I walked at a steady pace and acknowledged several in the audience as I whispered a "Hello" to a few familiar faces. Before I knew it, there I was near the altar. I particularly remember my Lafayette College friend Don Nikles giving me a thumbs up midway through the processional. That was a great confidence builder for me!

As we had rehearsed the night before, I gave my daughter a kiss and I shook hands with Erik and quietly said, "Congratulations." I took my place alongside my wife in the first-row pew. My wife knew my feelings, and she whispered, "YOU DID IT!"

Like instant replay, I ran the processional experience through my mind several times. For the veteran Parkinsonin, it was the triumph of a lifetime!

The standard pew helped me as far as standing and sitting were concerned. I simply pulled myself up by the back of the stall in front of me. I wasn't too sure where Raymond had positioned my walker. I tried to explore any options I might have as far as returning to the back of the church was concerned.

Following the opening prayer, I was particularly interested in hearing Cinnie's brother John Baldwin read from the Bible, namely I Corinthians 12.31–38. As expected, John's delivery was flawless as he employed the appropriate intonations and pauses to drive home the message from the scriptures.

When it came to communion, I felt I should have participated for Father Lew's sake. However, I was nervous about the route prescribed and so I hesitated, and before I knew it, the communion phase was completed.

Finally, there was my daughter Priscilla's solo of the difficult song entitled *Evergreen,* which was popularized by Barbara Streisand. I admired Priscilla's courage for even trying to sing the haunting song, and she came through as expected, with a beautiful soft rendition of the melody. The key to the delivery is the soloist's holding of the final note for several bars, and Priscilla sang the ending perfectly. Immediately upon hearing Priscilla wrap up the last note, her boyfriend Rob rose in the audience and led a round of applause.

Soon after, Alison and Erik were in an embrace and kissing, symbolizing their status as man and wife. After a round of applause to acknowledge the existence of Mr. & Mrs. Erik B. Swift, the organist started the recession. Again I faced the aisle, this time in reverse. Relieved that the ordeal was over, I decided to enjoy myself and I shook hands with many well-wishers as I strode back down the aisle. At the end of the line, I spotted my walker and positioned it so that I could conveniently meet everyone in the congregation as they exited.

The utter joy of the occasion was expressed on everyone's face as they shook my hand and, in some cases, introduced themselves. There were many surprises, such as Mrs. Lloyd Dille—the widow of my mentor at Halsey Stuart & Co.—who easily must have been eighty-five years old. I also enjoyed meeting some of Alison's coworkers, all of whom mentioned that they enjoyed working with Alison. Since I had posted the acceptances as they rolled in, many of the names were familiar and it was fun to match names with faces upon introduction.

Given the time gap between the wedding and the reception—approximately three hours—most of the attendees were in no hurry to complete the formality of the reception line. I was so wrapped up in meeting all the people that I completely lost track of time. As the line finally ended, everyone had moved outside and I was left alone inside the church lobby. I could feel a slight tightness developing in my body. I wanted to go to the bathroom quickly before I had trouble negotiating my unfamiliar tuxedo zipper, somewhat blocked by the purely decorative cummerbund, because of an impending freeze-up. I wasn't even sure where the bathroom was!!

Nancy Swift, the mother of the groom, appeared on the scene and she noticed my discomfort. She led me to the men's room, where I dismantled the tuxedo sufficiently to relieve myself. Afterward, Nancy helped me battle the stairs and find my wife in her car. Although we were slated to proceed immediately to the hotel for a photo shoot, Cinnie and I decided to take a break and rest at our home before heading to the hotel. I wanted to clear up the rigidity and give a new round of medicine a chance to take effect. We telephoned ahead to tell the wedding party to start the photo session without us.

We relaxed and caught our breath for almost an hour. The football scores produced some pleasant surprises, as Lafayette rolled over Holy Cross by a score of 56–20, and Bucknell pummeled Colgate 41–7. With Lehigh victorious over Fordham, the ensuing Lafayette versus Lehigh game would be for more than the year's bragging rights. For the first time since 1994, the L–L game would be for the Patriot League title and an automatic berth in the NCAA Division I-AA playoffs.

Around six p.m., Cinnie and I left for the Madison Hotel. When we arrived, we were immediately greeted by my sister and the entire Wenzel family delegation (approximately six strong). John Wenzel challenged me to play the piano, and so I obliged with one song, a ballad from the 1950s entitled *Teach Me Tonight* and recorded on Columbia Records by Jo Stafford. Soon, the entire wedding photo session was centered around the piano. The professional photographer coached us through several poses and, at long last, he announced the pre-reception phase of photos was over. Within moments, the cocktail hour began.

Everyone at the reception seemed anxious to line up some hors d'oeuvres for me or to fetch me a cocktail. I appreciated the courtesy, but my hands were not the steadiest. As a result, I began spilling my chardonnay all over my tux. My Lafayette friends, some seventeen strong, were all excited about the sudden emergence of our alma mater as a Patriot League football power, not to mention the upcoming game against Lehigh. Their enthusiasm led to even more spillage. I took my food in smaller increments and I believe I was much neater food-wise. I positioned my walker in the foyer of the reception area, and it seemed that almost everyone passed my station.

When the lights blinked, I realized it was time for the cocktail party to end and the main reception to begin. Soon, the maitre d'hotel—Tim McHale—was lining up the wedding party for a grand march into the main ballroom. The lead-off members were to be the parents of the bride followed by the parents of the groom. Each one of us would be separately announced over the public address system. As the preliminaries to the march-in stretched on a bit, I began to feel a little shaky and I had to alert Tim to expedite the process if he wanted to see me in action. He responded very quickly, and the band closed off their song and broke into a drum-roll indicating that the wedding party would soon be introduced to the masses! Indeed, Cinnie and I were announced first and we strolled across the dance floor to our appointed table. Kelly Dodson had set my walker in place, so I could sit down the second I arrived at the table. Again, I had traversed a modest area, under pressure, without any outside assistance.

The remainder of the wedding party was dutifully announced and received the roaring approval of the audience. The initial activity after the wedding party was in place was the traditional first dance of the newly created husband and wife team of Alison and Erik. The couple selected the classic Sinatra ballad *I've Got You Under My Skin*. Soon, the band played a few transition notes and led into the Billy Joel favorite *I Like You Just the Way You Are*. I should have recognized my cue. As Alison approached my table, I knew it was time for me to dance. As we embraced and started to dance, I heard the approval of the crowd. As I gradually turned Alison to the point where I was facing two tables of Lafayette supporters, the entire delegation rose to its collective feet and applauded while cheering my efforts. It was like the greatest moment in my life!

Once I sat down, the tempo of the music increased dramatically. With my confidence and ego somewhat charged, I attempted to dance to some faster numbers. The will was there but my body just wouldn't cooperate. After a few minutes of rapid dancing, I decided to take a seat. No sense going crazy!

After a while, the band stopped playing to allow us time for dinner. As I watched the waiter at our table ladle out the soup course into some very flat soup plates, I envisioned myself struggling for hours with the tasty lobster bisque. I requested a mug from the waiter. The mug was just the answer, as I could consume my bisque without spilling or dripping any.

I was particularly proud of my new son-in-law and daughter when I noticed the miniature easel on our table. The easel contained a message from the newly-weds, which read:

Dear Family and Friends,

> *Thank you for celebrating our*
> *Wedding with us. Your presence*
> *Makes this day all the more joyous. In*
> *Lieu of favors, we are making a donation to*
> *The Parkinson's Disease Foundation,*
> *A cause which is near and dear to our hearts.*

> *With much love,*
> *Alison and Erik*

During the course of the evening, I mentioned to the official photographer that I wanted to obtain a large photograph of the Lafayette College delegation. I had hoped to capture this group without disrupting the entire event, but there were just too many of us! I made an announcement (along with news of the day's spectacular victory over Holy Cross) and assigned a place for the photograph. When assembled, the space just wasn't large enough and so we moved to the center of the dance floor. We also wanted to get Alison and Erik in the photo. We followed the cake cutting ceremony in the photographer's list of priorities. I hoped that the picture would be clear enough to submit to the forthcoming edition of the *Lafayette College Alumni News.* The back of the publication had a section dedicated to wedding pictures, and I was determined to have our wedding represented.

One by one, various friends of mine came and sat next to me and we reminisced about high school, college, work, or life in general. Many of the women invited me to dance, but I only dared a few. I think it was Fran Nikles who wore me out!

At approximately eleven-fifteen p.m., my bodily functions virtually shut down, and I knew that I was through for the night. I had given my all, and so I gave the signal to Kelly Dodson, who then pushed me all the way from the dance floor to Room 109. I was in bed before midnight, and slept soundly. The rest of the wedding activities involved only my limited participation, or so I thought, and I slept pretty well.

By seven the next morning, I had maneuvered my way to the hotel lobby, but I was a little nervous about trying the down slope of the handicapped ramp. Therefore, I set up camp near a table used for making phone calls and the like. Again, my former work friend Ed Ellingham was in the area, and he asked if I needed any help. I let him fetch me some coffee, juice, and a muffin. We chatted for a while and soon he was off on his morning jog. I wanted to return to the room and make sure my wife was stirring, because she was in charge of the wedding brunch that she was co-hosting with her brother John Baldwin. The brunch was slated to begin at ten a.m.

Around nine a.m., I received a telephone call from my friend Raymond, who apparently had volunteered his services to take some wedding guests to Newark Airport for their trip home. He was concerned that he might get lost, and so I said I would drive with him to the terminal. The round trip to the airport would be a little less than an hour, and so I figured I could just about make the wedding brunch on time.

Actually, I was just late enough for the brunch to be fashionably late, and I was welcomed with a polite cheer and some applause. I was pleased to sit with Erik and his parents. Also, I was glad to accommodate my promise to the Spences, who had made the trip from Williamsburg, Virginia. The night before, they were just starting to chat with me and I told them it was my bedtime, but that I would try to hook up with them at the brunch. Chris Spence was quite helpful in securing me a full plate of food, and we did a lot of reminiscing at the table.

My Lafayette College roommate, John Hickman, asked me if I needed any help, and I invited him back to Room 109 to help me pack, organize my tux for return, and just make sure I didn't forget anything before checking out by one p.m. (We had a one hour extension on our checkout.) The time with John also helped us organize our rendezvous for the Lafayette versus Lehigh game, which was closing in on us. Soon the best man, Scott Douglas, was knocking at our door, and he collected my tuxedo for return to the store in Hoboken. John helped me with anything heavy and had most of our bulky luggage organized near the door.

Given a free hour, I took the time to do my ordinary Parkinson's repetitive functions, such as refilling my pill carrying case. I had taken a few bonus pills on both Friday and Saturday to try and stem off any freeze-ups, and with few exceptions had done very well for the two-day period. Now I would begin the process of tapering off these special doses to comply with my daily routine. I contemplated a relaxing afternoon with my sister Betty and brother-in-law John Wenzel, along with my friend Raymond Monroe as we watched the New York Jets and the other NFL football teams in action. My wife, the consummate hostess, would ply us with hors d'oeuvres, lunch, and drinks. We all complained of having full stomachs, but somehow we had enough room for Cinnie's goodies.

Erik and Alison dropped by to take an accounting of their wedding gifts. They didn't realize, I don't think, that it would take three to four hours to inventory the mound of gifts and checks. At first the process was exhilarating, but soon the extensive detail seemed to wear out the newlyweds. They turned down our invitation for a light dinner at The Meeting Place in order to complete their project. Erik's schedule included a round trip to Hoboken sometime before the night was out. They envisioned little sleep before their five a.m. departure the next day. They were headed for a Hawaiian Honeymoon!

Other events of the evening:

- Mr Swift, father of the groom, suffers an aneurysm near the aorta heart valve . . . undergoes three hours of surgery after driving all the way from Madison to Toms River, New Jersey.
- Cinnie slips on the cellar stairs when the heel of her shoe breaks. Fortunately, Uncle John and I are close at hand to grab her and keep her from sliding all the way down the steps.
- Erik returns from Hoboken just in time to catch the pre-arranged taxi to Newark Airport. Alison mentions something to the effect that Erik al-

ways sleeps in his clothes. He could change clothes in Hawaii.
- Later in the week, Mr. Swift was taken out of intensive care and actually returned home by the end of the week.
- My sister and her husband John left our house early on Monday morning for lunch with my cousin Warren Hale. Their departure marked the end of the wedding events. It was time to organize the Lafayette versus Lehigh weekend, which would start in only four days.

A few weeks after the wedding, my friend John Menger called our house and I asked him,

"John, did you enjoy the wedding?"

John was quick to reply. "How could you not enjoy the wedding? It was the wedding of the century!"

From our lodging in Harrisburg, Pennsylvania, we allowed five hours travel time for a game that started at noon and was less than 100 miles away. We didn't want to miss a thing!

Chapter 11

Road Trips!!!

Project Iowa

As an avid football fan, I had always wanted to see a football game at Penn State University in State College, Pennsylvania. Named Beaver Stadium after one of its founding fathers, the stadium at PSU is massive and seats a capacity crowd of 108,062—the second largest capacity in the nation. Traditionally, the size of the stadium notwithstanding, the tickets are all sold out to season ticket holders, alumni, and friends, and only a modest allotment is made to the visiting team. In July 2004, I had asked Sam Stellatella, a former all-state (NJ) football player and a Nutley High School classmate of mine, about the modus operandi for obtaining tickets. I could have entered a lottery for tickets to the PSU versus Akron University game, but that game and the other one he suggested (Purdue) had conflicted with my obligations at Lafayette. Sam more or less indicated that tickets to any other PSU home games would be extremely hard to come by, probably impossible.

Kelly Dodson is a homegrown Iowa product, and his passion for Iowa University football is literally written on his sleeve. The date for the Iowa versus Penn State game was October 23, 2004, and when I asked Kelly if he would like to work on obtaining some tickets, he immediately expressed a let's-go-for-it attitude. The fact that this was Penn State's homecoming added to the challenge.

Kelly's first call was to the Iowa University Athletic Department, and he was quickly informed that the Hawkeyes' allotment had been spoken for well in advance. We were equally disappointed upon calling the Penn State ticket office. It seemed impossible to conceive how almost 110,000 tickets could disappear so quickly, especially in an area so sparsely populated as State College, Pennsylvania. We essentially gave up on the project as a lost cause. But then I had the idea of trying to use my handicapped condition as a means of securing three tickets to the game. We again called the Penn State ticket office, and they connected us this time with a special number that handled handicapped applicants. Upon rendering my New Jersey Disabled Person number, the sales representative indicated he could supply us with three tickets to the Iowa versus Penn State game. Additionally, he supplied us with a parking pass to the handicapped parking lot and an elevator ticket to the wheelchair area on the third floor. We were relieved to hear that the section was located underneath the upper tier of the stadium. We had only to supply a credit card number and three tickets to the game would be on the way to my house the next day! In a matter of a few minutes, we were done! A few days later, as promised, the tickets arrived in the mail along with the other documents for parking and the elevator.

"Project Iowa" was also perfectly timed as far as my responsibilities to my daughter's wedding arrangements were concerned. The date of the game—October 23—was also the one for my daughter's bridal shower to be held at my house. Some forty women would be descending upon my house, and we would be almost 200 miles away that day.

We dragged our feet a little bit in lining up a motel or hotel in the Penn State vicinity. Every potential lodging was completely booked for the weekend. Motel 8 in Lewistown, about thirty miles from the game, had two rooms available when we called, but when we called back within fifteen minutes, someone else had beaten us to the punch and reserved the rooms out from under us. We stretched our calling area out to Harrisburg, and we eventually settled on the Crowne Plaza Hotel in the State Capitol area. Soon our plans were solidified. We would set off from Chatham the Friday afternoon before the game, arrive in Harrisburg in time for dinner, and then get up early enough to set off for the Iowa–PSU game by seven a.m. We allowed five hours travel time for a game that started at noon and was less than 100 miles away. We didn't want to miss a thing!

The distances involved with "Project Iowa" would indeed be a challenge for any Parkinsonian. The trip, as described, entailed two three-hour components coming and two more on the way home. Sitting in a car that long is not the most comfortable situation, but Kelly, Raymond, and I amused each other with trivia games and the like. The time passed more quickly than I had anticipated. The connecting link on Route 322 between Harrisburg and Penn State was the only aggravating stretch.

Highway construction, a dense fog, and the heavy game traffic delayed us to the extent we traversed about five miles in one hour. But when the fog lifted, we were immediately blessed with a dose of colorful fall foliage. Following the PSU instruction handout, we found our way to the handicapped parking lot some 3.5 hours after leaving Harrisburg.

Before the trip and while driving to the game, I dreaded the thought of using one of the typical porta-John facilities that usually decorate the parking lots of major stadiums. Much to my surprise, the PSU version was immaculate and included railings appropriate for most handicapped situations. The unit was even wide enough for my walker to fit in with me. Also, the bathrooms inside the stadium walls were quite impressive, even beyond halftime of the game. Most public bathrooms at professional stadiums (Giants Stadium comes to mind) are fairly repulsive once the game gets under way.

Our parking spot was probably some 400 yards from the stadium entrance, equivalent to a modest length par four in golf. However, walking was unnecessary because the PSU plan included a jitney which continually drove passengers from the lot to Gate B of Beaver Stadium. Despite our Iowa gear (i.e., hats, jackets, etc.) the local PSU fans were polite and respectful of our loyalty to Iowa University. Once we were at the base of the stadium, we had to negotiate the security checkpoint. The security was thorough but moved along rapidly. I was amazed at how well I handled all the walking. Soon we arrived at our seats and we had a spectacular view of the entire stadium and the football field as well. A TV monitor would avail us of any replay observations and update us on the important Lafayette versus Fordham game.

The pre-game activity showcased the Penn State University marching band, which consumed almost the entire field when in formation. As the PSU students filed in, they each wore a white t-shirt, in most cases layered over a sweatshirt or long-sleeved turtleneck, and dark pants or dungarees. The entire stadium was a mass of white except for a ten-yard stretch of black and gold where the Iowa fans were seated. You could see the Iowa fans maneuvering their pom-poms and giving the appearance of making some cheers, but the cacophony emanating from the Penn State cheering section instantly drowned out the Iowans' efforts.

As soon as the National Anthem was completed, the right side of the crowd burst out cheering in perfect unison:

WE ARE

To which the left side responded equally as loud:

PENN STATE

The cheer persisted for several minutes and reverberated throughout the stadium. It was impossible to hear even the person sitting next to you.

On Iowa's first possession, it was obvious that the Penn State crowd was going to be a factor in determining the final score of the game. It was readily apparent that the Iowa quarterback could not audibly change the play at the line of scrimmage. His attempts to talk into the ears of his individual linemen and backs only intensified the noisy crowd. The stubborn PSU defense forced an Iowa punt and, as the crowd vocally endorsed the fourth down and eight situation, the Hawkeye snapper sailed the ball over his punter's head and on into the end zone. To avoid a possible Penn State touchdown, the Iowa punter kicked the ball over the endline, resulting in a "safety7" of two points for PSU.

Unfortunately for Penn State, the offense was totally ineffective against the strong Iowa defense. During the course of the game, the Nittany Lions could only muster two drives within enemy territory. Two field goal attempts were wide of the mark. Later on, with a few minutes left in the game, Iowa took a deliberate safety to narrow the score to 6–4 in their favor. The intense battle ended just that way. In my mind, the final score was Iowa 6, The Crowd 4. The local Harrisburg newspaper headline the next morning read:

6–4

2–5

UGH!!!!!!!!!

The press continued its assault on veteran coach Joe Paterno. Although he was the second winningest coach in collegiate history, he had sustained three losing seasons in the past four years. The loss to Iowa put his mid-season record at 2–5 and 0–3 in the Big Ten. At the age of seventy-seven, he was criticized for lack of imagination on offense. The futility of the once proud Nittany Lions was expressed in its production of just six first downs and no points for the entire game. At the college level, we were surprised by the chorus of boos which seemed to follow every aborted PSU third-down play. The normally supportive crowd was undoubtedly expressing its dissatisfaction with Paterno's coaching more than with the players' performance.

Despite the ugly score, the game was truly intense and interesting to watch. "Project Iowa" was indeed a success, and I felt a sense of accomplishment for all we had done. Even the hotel accommodations in Harrisburg were marvelous.

The trip to Penn State can be construed as a form of physical therapy. My Parkinson's related freeze-ups subsided in number and intensity. The trip illustrated to me the advantage of being socially active and simply keeping moving as much as possible. Upon our return to Chatham, we started planning our next major excursion. We started to lay the groundwork for a 2006 trip to West Lafayette, Indiana, home of the Purdue Boilermakers and possibly a game at Iowa's home stadium against Illinois.

Actually, our late November road trip to Newark, Delaware for Lafayette's first participation in the I-AA playoffs was gratifying, though the game ended in a loss. In the game's closing minutes, as Lafayette drove toward the tying (or conceivably go-ahead) score, the Pard's fumbled on the Delaware 18-yard line and the Blue Hens turned the miscue into a two-touchdown lead. We were so close. A strong returning cast for next year gave us hope that we would again have a shot at the national title.

The Georgia Tech Basketball Game

When I first checked out the Lafayette men's basketball schedule for 2004–2005, I was surprised to see two major powerhouses on our schedule. In addition to

Louisville University, Lafayette would also challenge Georgia Tech in the upcoming season. Tech was one of the major surprises of the 2003–2004 college basketball season, finishing in second place in the NCAA March Madness tournament in March. While Tech rolled to the number-two slot in the nation, Lafayette College was eliminated in the first round of the Patriot League tournament and ended its season with a theoretically successful 18–10 record. But they also endured five straight conference losses. Although a classic mismatch between LC and Georgia Tech loomed, I felt it might be interesting to follow the team to Atlanta and see how they would fare against the highly ranked Wramblin' Wreck. That the game was being played between Christmas and the new year would help my wife relieve some of the holiday stress. My pal Raymond said he was interested in the contest, and so we had a mini-entourage.

Tickets to the game would probably be available, I thought, in view of the Georgia Tech home facility (the Alexander Memorial Coliseum) having a seating capacity of 9,191. But upon checking the local ticket office in Atlanta, I discovered that all of Georgia Tech's basketball games were sold out pre-season, and that no general admission tickets were available. I then tried the Lafayette College ticket office to see if Lafayette received any allotment for the game, but no tickets were available. I then called Coach Fran O'Hanlon, and he confirmed my fears of the ticket situation at Tech. He said that his department received a token allotment for college officials and parents of players. If any of this package were available, he indicated he would save me some. After a short waiting period, I received a phone call from Coach O'Hanlon indicating that he could provide me with four tickets to the Lafayette–Georgia Tech basketball game on December 28, 2005 at the Alexander gym. He immediately mailed the tickets to me.

Tickets in hand, I set out to line up flights and hotel and dinner reservations for the time around the date of the game. Raymond and I took out a directory of Atlanta motels and searched for one where the windows opened in the rooms (one of my wife's general requirements).

Cinnie also wanted a hotel located in the upscale Buckhead area of Atlanta. This entailed more telephoning than expected, but eventually we landed upon the Sheraton Buckhead (nee The Terrace Garden Hotel). Raymond arranged for a room with a mini-balcony for a relatively inexpensive rate of $109 per night. A mid-day flight on Continental Airlines the day before the game seemed to provide a comfortable time to fly.

We booked the convenient flight and at the same time we ordered wheelchairs to assist me through the Newark and Atlanta airports.

As the date of the game approached, I deduced that we would be on the same flight as the Lafayette basketball team! Marty Zippel, a fellow member of the LC Maroon Club, and Phil LaBella (assistant director of athletic communications) would also be on the same flight. On the relatively crowded airplane, the tall members of the Lafayette basketball team seemed even larger, in some cases massive (e.g., Jamal Douglas).

At approximately noon on Tuesday, the day of the Tech game, we watched the team go through its preliminary shoot-around at the Alexander gym. The fourteen members of the Lafayette traveling team were divided into two seven-man squads, with the seven most active players wearing maroon shirts and the second team wearing white jerseys. Coach O'Hanlon worked his players through some light drills, emphasizing ball movement and rebounding positioning.

While we watched the Leopards practice, we were somewhat awed by the Georgia Tech gym. Alexander Coliseum resembles a huge circular sugar bowl with the lower two-thirds of the structure lying below ground. We estimated the location of our tickets, and we knew our seats were on courtside or floor level. At first glance, there was no access to this level except via the stairs, which made about a thirty-row drop. I was not looking forward to making that move! For myself and other handicapped fans, the method of gaining access to the seats without inflicting injury created a real challenge.

The only arena personnel on duty at noontime were kitchen workers readying the heavy load of snack equipment for that evening. We would have to plan on getting to the Coliseum early so that we could negotiate the stairway hurdle.

The team was soon off the court and heading toward the Grand Hyatt Regency Hotel, and we decided to follow them back to their temporary quarters. The hotel lobby features a spectacular array of balconies that extend skyward up the full height of the structure. The elevator resembles a tubular spaceship and is visible from all four sides. It operates from the innermost point of the building. The very top of the hotel has a rotating bar, which pivots 360 degrees to enable patrons to get a full view of the Atlanta skyline. A massive dining room, several cocktail lounges with massive TV sets, and a plethora of gift shops round out the lower floors of the Hyatt.

But the Hyatt seems to reflect the problems of down-town Atlanta. Once the center of social activities, the core of Atlanta had migrated toward Buckhead and other areas. When we assumed a table for four in the dining room, we were the only group dining there. Then Marty Zippel, Lafayette Hall of Fame basketball player and one of the first LC cagers to score 1,000 points in his career, joined our table. When the Lafayette College Maroon Club voted on its top fifteen athletes of the twentieth century to commemorate the arrival of the year 2000, Marty was among those selected.

Although eighty-one years old, Marty maintained an active role in supporting the Lafayette basketball team. He attended most all of the school's games (home and away) and was on hand for many of the team's practices. On this particular day, he expressed some disappointment that John Feinstein, one of the nation's premier sports writers, had omitted his name in his most recent work, the biography of "Red" Auerbach. Marty was a Celtic in the late 1940s, and he had some newspaper clippings to prove his role in the lineup. The press referred to him as Baby Doll Zippel, in recognition of his youthful appearance. While visiting with us in Atlanta, Zippel also reviewed his decision to play for Lafayette even though he was actively recruited by national powers such as Southern California and Notre Dame. Zippel's mother was ill at the time of his release from the air force, and Marty didn't want to stray too far from the Easton area.

Having a session with Marty was a real treat. He seemed somewhat optimistic that the new President of Lafayette—David Weiss—would lean toward favoring scholarships for basketball, thus putting us on par with the other Patriot League colleges. But soon Marty had to leave our group because he was slated to eat a pre-game lunch with the team at three p.m.

While we finished lunch, Coach O'Hanlon stopped by our table and encouraged us to cheer loudly for the Leopards. After lunch, my college fraternity brother Ted Gailer, a resident of suburban Atlanta (Alpharetta), gave us a tour of the greater Atlanta environs. When we returned to the Sheraton Buckhead, we still had about an hour to kill, and so we taught Ted how to play Skip-Bo. The time flew by quickly and soon it was six p.m. Although the distance to the Alexander gym was relatively short, we could be sure that Atlanta rush hour traffic plus the compression of fans filing into the Georgia Tech arena would be fairly intense.

We were somewhat banking on the handicapped sticker, which I had brought from my car in New Jersey, to guide us by the traffic and position us close to the arena. But by six-fifteen p.m., all the handicapped slots had been taken and we had to use parking spots on the street, which took us, it seemed, several miles from the stadium. Ted volunteered to drop us off at the gate and to find a spot somewhere within walking distance of the gym. As we unloaded his car, including my rollader (four-wheel walker with a seat), a Tech official approached Ted and started pointing to a make-shift parking slot just a few feet from the entrance to the arena. Ted quickly snagged the spot before the official changed his mind. I pointed out that I thought the official resembled Bobby Crimmens (legendary Tech coach from the 1980s and 1990s), with his youthful face and brilliant white hair.

We entered the gym about thirty minutes before game time. We quickly summoned an usher, who we hoped would guide us to our seats down on the floor, some thirty rows below. It really disappointed us that the ushers with security badges sewn onto their uniforms didn't know where the elevator that could take us directly to the floor was.

Because the usher crew was so lacking in information, we again resorted to the kitchen personnel who had helped us at midday. Finally we found the elevator, but it could not be used until the basketball floor was cleared of all the players. An attractive middle-aged female usher sensed our problem and said she would line us up with the appropriate contacts to gain admission to the playing floor. Sure enough, the instant that the Tech and Lafayette players had completed their drills and were seated in their respective courtside seats, she signaled Ted and the rest of our group to hop on the elevator to floor level.

The narrow aisleway of ninety-six feet or so that we had to traverse to get to our seats was filled with gym bags, water bottles, warm-up jerseys, and a mass of communications wires that were part of the TV and radio connections pertaining to the game. We soon passed Dick Hammer and his wife (his main spotter), who have been broadcasting Lafayette sporting events for thirty-eight years for WEST-AM, the local Easton, Pennsylvania radio station. As we approached our seats, it felt like everyone in the stands was watching us negotiate all the nuances and barriers along the way. Just as the public address announcer was about to dramatically present the starting lineups, we arrived at the four seats in Row CC, the tickets for which Fran O'Hanlon had mailed us some months ago. At long last, we were ready to watch some basketball!

Although Lafayette upset the Notre Dame basketball team in 1988, few if any local fans held much hope for the Leopards as they faced the nationally ranked (#9) Georgia Tech Yellow Jackets. In the 2003–2004 season, Tech had finished 28–10 and wound up second in the NCAA Tourney. At year-end, Georgia Tech was the second best team in the nation! Meanwhile, Lafayette finished fifth in the Patriot League, whose league champion (Lehigh University) had to try to win their play-in game to be one of the Final 64. Lehigh lost the play-in game to Florida A&M.

But this was another year and hopes were starting to evolve, showing that Lafayette might have improved over the summer months. Starting slow in 2004, they had just defeated an athletic California University (Northridge) team in overtime. And most Lafayette supporters felt the team had one of the best coaches in the nation in Fran O'Hanlon. Also, the Patriot League had perhaps advanced a notch, as represented by Bucknell's back-to-back victories over St. Joseph's and Pitt.

The game started with Tech grabbing the opening center jump, and they were the first to score. However, Lafayette stayed with the Jackets and was partly inspired by seven-foot senior captain Jamie Hughes' first three-point field goal in his career at Lafayette. Baskets by Bilal Abdullah and Andre Capusan gave LC its last lead of the game at 11–10. By halftime, the Pards were still hanging around, with a score of 37–29. The last flicker of hope came in a brief third quarter rally by the Pards that brought the score to 49–43 with thirteen minutes left in the game. But then Anthony Morrow, a six foot, five inch freshman guard for Tech, exploded on a three-point tear. Soon the entire Tech team was scoring at will and the game got away from Lafayette. There was no stopping the Wreck; they went on a 27–3 scoring streak to quickly dash the courageous underdogs. The final read: GT 92, LC 58.

As the Lafayette players lined up for the traditional handshakes with the opposing players, the small contingency of Leopard supporters gave their team a rousing round of applause. Despite the appearance of the final score, the fans from Lafayette would not soon forget how competitive the Pards were for two-thirds of the game.

Reversing our tracks to the elevator and back to ground level was much smoother than our trip earlier in the evening. We waited for the rest of the 9,000 fans to leave the arena, and then we had a clear path to our privileged parking spot arranged by the Bobby Crimmens look alike.

Other road trips of modest length included an excursion to Marist College in Poughkeepsie, New York, and to Bucknell University in Lewisberg, Pennsylvania. Bucknell gave us a preview of its power with a 70–34 thrashing of LC. The Bison eventually captured the Patriot League Tourney and shocked the basketball pundits with an upset of Kansas University in the first round of the NCAA. Holy Cross' win over Notre Dame in the first round of the NIT added to the Patriot League being a rising force to be reckoned with. The successful victories of the two schools also put pressure on the Lafayette administration to revamp its position on scholarships.

Chapter 12

What Lies Ahead?

You may want to skip this chapter. Perhaps I have saved the worst for last.

It is very easy to get discouraged as a Parkinson's patient. Some mornings, when it takes so long to get dressed, when it takes such an effort to lift myself off the bed, negative thoughts sometimes creep into my head and I feel like just throwing in the towel. As I ruminate on the inevitability of my degeneration, I am reminded that matters can only get worse, not better. The only way to sustain any kind of lifestyle is to take more pills. Given my physical condition and age, the neurologists at Columbia have indicated that I already have been at or near a peak load for my pill schedule. Barring any imminent pill discoveries on the research front, it appears I can carry on in perpetual struggle or I can take a risk—hopefully a minimal risk—and undergo the brain cell surgery. My family and close friends are not too enamored with the "brain implant" option.

Sometimes I can block such thoughts from my mind. What brings them into focus is when something goes wrong or results in a visible embarrassment. For example, when I left to hit golf balls a few weeks ago, I sensed that my limbs were a bit off, but I was hoping that by the time I got to the driving range I would be regaining the on slot and be able to hit balls with some authority. After I found an appropriate station, I poured my entire pail of balls into the tray adjoining the tee. I usually advanced five or six balls at a time onto the mat. As I lined myself to hit some five irons, I could hardly move. I hit one ball, a feeble grounder about thirty yards, and when I addressed my second effort, I realized I was totally frozen. My feet felt like they weighed a thousand pounds, like huge cement blocks locked into the ground. I tried to adjust them to get a better address to the ball, but I just couldn't move them. So I put some sort of swing on the ball, and again barely hit it thirty yards.

To top matters off, the experience was somewhat socially embarrassing to me. Phillip Ng is one of my friends from the Lafayette Maroon Club executive committee, and coincidentally he was on the premises of the range performing his proper role as a salesman for the Addidas Corporation. After completing his call on the local pro shop, he stopped by to watch Doug and me hit some golf balls. Although Phil was aware that I had PD, he had never seen the degree to which it could affect my activities. Phil, a fantastic athlete in his own right (for twelve years he held almost all the LC pass reception statistics), showed an expression of compassion for my condition. It saddened me that I saddened him. I guess up to the day of this incident, I had only worked with Phil within the friendly confines of a boardroom.

But Phil had to get back to work. Meanwhile, I was also having difficulty gripping the club. Soon I tried to cradle the club in my left hand, then I swung my right arm in an arc-like manner until it landed on the top of my left hand and enabled me to form a somewhat improvised version of the traditional overlapping golf grip on the club. Although my swing was limited, the methodology of attaining a "flying" grip helped pull my psyche into the game.

I hit one more ball, maybe a hundred yards or so, and I decided to sit down and rest my knees and back. As I sat on the wall separating my hitting area from my friend Doug Hobby's, I tried to analyze what was wrong with me. Usually, golf or any physical activity overrode the Parkinson's factor for me. But on this particular day, I just couldn't will an effective golf swing. As I looked at my feet, I made the assessment that possibly the rubber soles on my shoes were creating overwhelming friction with the substance covering the driving tee. I mentioned this to Doug, and he seemed to agree. He quickly rescued my golf shoes from the car and I tried those on. I felt better as soon as I had them on, and soon I was out there hitting balls straight and quite a bit further. To Doug's surprise, I hit all the balls in the bucket.

During this time period, though, I became quite discouraged with my future. The day before the driving range incident, I suddenly froze at the radio repair shop. It took me forever to write a check to the dealer. This was at a time of day that was usually pretty favorable for me (eleven-fifteen a.m.). Consistency in behavior patterns was breaking down throughout the Paul A. Luscombe universe.

The best time (i.e., the best on positions) occurred approximately twenty-five to thirty minutes after my opening salvo of four pills: 2 corba doba, 1 comtan, and 1 mirapex. From six a.m. to almost nine a.m., I was just about invincible, or at least I felt that way! As the day wore on, though, each succeeding on period was shorter than the prior period, and around evening time, my standard on unit had compressed to two hours. When possible, I began to skip those social events that took place in the evening and saved my social efforts for luncheons and afternoon golf.

For years while under the grip of Parkinson's disease, I had maintained an active social and athletic schedule. Though imperfect, pill management worked and I could take bonus pills on evenings when I was out among my coworkers or friends.

Also, in the past, my off periods were not so debilitating. I could still make my way to the door or the bathroom, though it was often a struggle. My hands would cramp slightly, but now they get totally useless. My experience at the driving range was typical of this process. I could always manufacture some sort of swing that enabled me to hit the ball somewhat straight. Now I was afraid I might become a menace on the course with one of my sideway shots. A number of my shanks—it makes me nervous just looking at the word—hit the side wall of my hitting cubicle during my ill-fated practice session. I surmised that for future rounds, if I locked myself into one of these power freezes, I would remain in the golf cart for a few holes rather than risk injuring one of my fellow players. In addition to his other problems, the PD golfer with a case of the shanks is a miserable individual.

What has been most affected over the years is my balance. I am now consciously aware of the risk of falling, whereas a few years ago, I rarely thought about not being able to control my body's actions. It was simply second nature. Reverting to the above golfing example, I felt that I might fall down when I exercised the torque implicit in the normal golf swing as I brought the club through the ball. And so I cut the swing down to a minimum pivot, which inhibited my power potential but at least kept me standing on both my feet!

On the coordination scale, golf ranks as one of the most difficult activities. For almost all golfers, balance is axiomatic and is not something you work on every day. I, however, have to protect against falling over, and this overrides any other focal points when I am trying to execute the swing.

Since the middle of 2003, at least four factors seemed to reverse my otherwise good feelings about myself.

- First, I attempted to address my "bad knee" problem with a back operation labeled a non-invasive procedure. My back was fixed up fairly well, but I still suffer from a knee that permanently throbs and feels like it is sprained.
- Second, the discontinuance of the "miracle drug" research program at Columbia due to the effect on the brains of rats. The drug seemed to soften the impact of freeze-ups and enabled me to extend my day when appropriate.
- Third, there was the closing of the physical therapy unit of Nova Care in Livingston. The main personnel have scattered and I have been unable to reattach with them.

- Fourth, since my appendectomy, I have been reluctant to start a new physical therapy program. Now that several months have passed, I intend to start a three-week program to hopefully improve my balance. (Program eventually started with MARA in Morristown; see chapter on Physical Therapy).

(The following paragraph was written randomly while I was in the off position. I did not edit the paragraph, hoping to illustrate how stifling the PD process can be.)

    Very little in the entire dialogue of the ON- OFF manuscript has been written about experiences involgling tne "OFF" positioin iof a PD victim;s day. First of all, almost by definition, the OFF po sition entails alck of obody movement and the abilityi to t ype or write. Keys are tough to keep from repeating, my glasses slide down my nose uncontrollably, and IK tend to just stare ou8t in space r atrher than stain myseof bt ty0ing. I twitch my feet and bodhy iu hopes that the recent medicine will "kick in". Once my hands are p laced on thecompuyter board, i8t is hard to take them offQ I must taje a little

    break between sentencews—each one requires great amounts of effort, I mustr tplace te kieyboard lower and closoer ti my body. My hands jus twont functiuon at a hihigher oevel . . . e. As I hink of all the work on my agenda,, this time loss aggravates me . . . A modest headache also annoys me. AHA! I start to regain some feeling in my hands and I elevate the keyboard to the full desk position. As I peruse the paragraph that I just wrote while in the "OFF" position, I can see the evidence of my difficulty as illustrated by the number of words underscored in red. I am almost back ON and I can continue writing about matters outlined in my Table of Contents for "Pills, Bills & Parkinson Disease"—Coping with the "OFF and ON" Syndrome.

(Actually, I have a theory that the typing actually helps restore my on stature more quickly. Although the first few sentences are a struggle, the slight wrist-finger-hand motions seem to be better reducers of the rigidity than some more physical tactics.)

As you have read this book, you probably noted several contradictions or statements reversed in subsequent chapters. This phenomenon arises because I write down the experiences when they happen, and my behavioral patterns are constantly changing over time.

In closing, as I analyze my fate, I am not overjoyed at the prospects of another ten years or so locked into this PD routine. But let's face it, most of us who survive to live in the sixty-five- to seventy-five-year-old age bracket have some sort of health limitation anyway! Arthritis, Alzheimer's, cancer, heart failure, prostate problems, hearing problems—the list goes on and on—all these ailments affect the aging component of our society. The members of my family, the members of the Chatham Mens Club, the members of the Class of 1960 at Lafayette, all these sectors of my life seem to want me to hang around a bit longer.

Maybe another wedding will get me motivated!